I0027372

SOLVING LIFESTYLE DISEASE WITH LIFESTYLE

First published in Australia in 2017 by Lu Behavioural Medicine Institute

3/89 Nelson Rd, Box Hill North, VIC 3129, Australia

National Library of Australia Cataloguing-in-Publication entry

Creator: Lu, Mingfu, author.
Title: Solving Lifestyle Disease with Lifestyle / Dr Mingfu Lu.
ISBN: 978-0-646-98340-0
Notes: Includes index.
Subjects: Nutritionally induced diseases-Prevention.
            Diet therapy.
            Sugar-free diet – Recipes.
            Blood sugar monitoring.

Cover design by X-colour studio.

Printed in Australia by Compass Printing Pty Ltd.

10 9 8 7 6 5 4 3 2 1

Disclaimer: The information contained in this book is provided for general purposes only. It is not intended as and should not be relied upon as medical advice. The publisher and authors are not responsible for any specific health needs that may require medical supervision. If you have underlying health problems, or have any doubts about the advice contained in this book, you should contact a qualified medical, dietary or other appropriated professional.

Solving Lifestyle Disease with Lifestyle

Mingfu Lu, PhD

Preface

For more than ten years, we have conducted heavy research, and finally received innumerable great achievements in return. Thousands and thousands of obese patients who also suffer from Triple H (hypertension, hyperlipidaemia, hyperglycaemia) benefit from our treatments. Of which, not only obese patients have lost weight and been back to their normal sizes, but also Triple H patients have reduced or even gotten rid of substance dependence. Because we have helped them to regain health and even rebuild wonderful lives, we have reaped blessings and appreciation. We have discovered the values of our lives from them, so we feel content and happy.

However, there is a sharp contrast between the recovered patients and others, who are greater in number: the majority of the society does not believe. Almost all of the doctors do not think it is possible. Where we have devoted the most efforts and time in the past, not to consult about treatments, but to persuade patients into believing that the results will be amazing, so their curiosity will be aroused and they might have a try. The real difficulty of work in the future is not the disease itself, but is people's ideological obstacle when facing the so-called 'lifelong disease', which was falsely formed in the past medical practice. How can we make more people to believe in the existence of such an 'unbelievable' new method faster? How to make not only tens of thousands of people, but also hundreds of thousands of people, millions of people, tens of millions of people, hundreds of millions of people, to have a try and benefit from it earlier? We feel the intense pressure but also responsibilities from this heavy workload. So, we have decided to write a book aimed to teach people, who would then teach other, to help hundreds of millions of patients of lifestyle disease and potential patients, and to initiate tens of thousands of elites of the generation to the solution of the issue. The progress of the issue can be accelerated thanks to the intelligence of the elites.

Our research is not solely based on existing medical theories, but more importantly, we have two basic medical beliefs. First, we believe that the actual aim of medical science is to follow human nature. Secondly, we believe the main means of following human instincts is live the right way.

We have made breakthroughs on the current existing medical theories based on a lot of medical practices. On the basis of practices, we have put forward 'Wisdom Model of Behavioural Health' which is a brand new concept in the medical field; not only that, we have also published 'Energy Conversion Theory', which is a bold investigation on the medical theory; and established 'Cell Comprehensive Revitalisation Program', which provides an effective solution for lifestyle disease in every different perspective.

The book is the footprints of the fight of Team 'Doctor Lu'. 'Solving Lifestyle Disease with Lifestyle' is not only a book, but it is a project of the generation, which cannot be done by the power of only one person. 'Doctor Lu' is not just one person, but a team. There are not only professional men, but also non-professionals. Some of them are beneficiaries, scattered among various industries. They are not confined to improve themselves, but rather the entire society. They contribute to this project by influencing the people around. Some of them make the project as their own goals. They devote a lot of valuable time and even precious emotion into this project. The team is still growing and expanding. Life is a journey of discovery. People make self-discoveries on the way of discovering the world. Life is a journey of achieving. They achieve their meaning in life on the way to achieving their goals.

The book is about natural human instinctive behaviour, rather than lifestyle disease. We sincerely hope that what the readers understand from this book is about human instincts, which is also the most central concept of the book. We mention Alternative Medicine Treatment because we have to point out that the main issue of the treatment is that it ignores human innate behaviour; we suggest new medical models, because we want to lead medicine back to revolving around instincts; we also mention cells to help people to understand 'instinct' more deeply; we have mentioned nutrition and exercise, this is because we are explaining that the basic idea of every means is 'follow our instincts'; we have given many real cases as examples, because all medical miracles are based on human instinct. Finally, we hope what you get from the book is to believe in potential abilities.

The targeted readers of this book are every single one of the patients with lifestyle disease, as well as the practitioners of health industry. The contents that are marked with 'selective reading for patients, compulsory reading for practitioners' are for practitioners, it discusses theories to great details. If general public has difficulty in understanding the contents, you can skim over it. If you are interested in it, you can do some advanced studies in it.

Contents

Contents

Chapter Three: Fight between Two Medical Models
(Selective Reading for Patients, Compulsory Reading for Practitioners)

Section One: Rethink Old Medical Thinking - 'Biomedical Model'

Section Two: Put Forward New Medical Thinking – Wisdom Model of Behavioural Health

Chapter Four: Amazing Effects Bring Out Theoretical Innovation

Section One: Amazing Effects, Novel Theories.

Section Two: Reason for Getting Lifestyle Disease Is Change in Energy Path.

Section Three: How Obesity Evolves Into Triple H and CCVD (Cardiac-Cerebral Vascular Disease)

Contents

Chapter Five: Self-Healing of Lifestyle Disease Using Human Instincts

Chapter Six: Nutrition and Exercise Are Main Means of Rehabilitation

Contents

Contents

Part One: Theory

Chapter One: Lifestyle Disease and Its Hazards

Section One: Menacing Lifestyle Disease

I.What Is 'Lifestyle Disease'?

When old friends meet, they will say, 'Long time no see, I see you have put on some weight'. The other party answers, 'Indeed, I have gained ten kilograms. I had a check-up that day, and doctor said I have got new disease: Hyperlipidaemia. What about you?' The other one says: 'It is a common disease – 'Triple H'! The doctor said if it could not be well controlled, and if it develops further, it will become cardiovascular disease!'

In recent years, with the continuous improvement in standard of living, obesity, 'Triple H' and cardiovascular disease have become phrases which are frequently mentioned when people talk about health. These types of diseases are different development phases of metabolic disease. Generally speaking, the symptoms of early stage of the disease are overweight and obesity; metaphase is developed to 'Triple H', namely hypertension, hyperlipidaemia and hyperglycaemia (diabetes); more severely, it will become cardiovascular disease in the later stage.

This type of disease is neither inherent (occasionally with genetic factors), nor bacterial or caused by virus infection. The diseases mostly come from unhealthy lifestyle. It is 'rich man's disease' derived from modern civilisation. We collectively call it as 'lifestyle disease'.

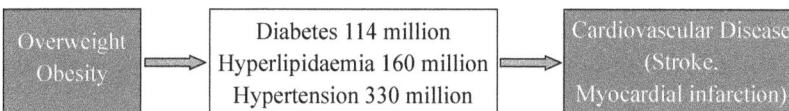

Overweight Obesity	Diabetes 114 million Hyperlipidaemia 160 million Hypertension 330 million	Cardiovascular Disease (Stroke, Myocardial infarction)

II. Early Deaths of Elites

China's Health Minister, Zhu Chen, said in the 66th Session of United Nations General Assembly High-level Meeting on the 'Prevention and Control of Noncommunicable Disease', 'Non-communicable diseases have become the leading health threat for Chinese people, accounting for 85% of death causes of population. Namely, when we are actively responding to infectious diseases, for example, AIDS, tuberculosis and malaria, non-communicable diseases (also known as lifestyle disease as we mentioned) have crept into the crowd and become number one health problem for Chinese people.'

Statistics show that cardiovascular disease kill up to three million people every year, more than thirty times as many as the death toll in Wenchuan Earthquake (killed ninety thousand people). Compared to devastating natural disasters, the attacks of cardiovascular disease to human are silent but rapid. Instead of having effective control with the development of modern medicine, the incidence of cardiovascular disease is rising year by year.

Lifestyle disease is everywhere. In terms of only entrepreneur group, cases of which entrepreneurs dying young due to cardiovascular disease can be found everywhere. Fox example:

In July 2001, Zuoyi Peng, General Manager of Tsingtao Brewery Group, suddenly suffered from myocardial infarction when swimming at the age of 56.

In March 2004, Kai Hu, General Manager of Beijing Dazhong Electric Appliance Co., Ltd., died of a heart attack at the age of 52.

In September 2005, CEO of Netease, Dedi Sun, suffered from sudden death at the age of 38.

In January 2006, Min Nan, Chairman of Shanghai Zhongfa Group, died of acute cerebral thrombosis at the age of 37.

In July 2008, Shengyu Zhang, Chairman of Tongrentang, had a heart attack at the age of 39.

In May 2012, Chuanyang Li, Vice General Manager of Jianghuai Automotive Company, had sudden cardiac death at the age of 49.

In November 2012, Yang Luo, Project Leader for J-15 carrier-based aircraft development had acute myocardial infarction at the age of 51.

In December 2012, Bo Sun, Vice President of PetroChina, died of cerebral hemorrhage at the age of 52.

......

As seen from the data investigated by Ciming Check-up Group, the average age of entrepreneurs who died from cardiovascular disease is 48. Most painfully, the age when they died was during their prime of life.

This is only in the business circles. There are countless people in art and literary circles who died of cardiovascular disease. Of which, there are persons who we know well:

Famous crosstalk performer, Yaowen Hou died of myocardial infarction at the age of 59.

Famous comedy actor, Xiumin Gao died of heart disease at the age of 46.

Yue Gu, actor, impersonator of Mao Zedong, died of myocardial infarction at the age of 68.

Famous playwright, Zuo Liang (main founder of sitcom I Love My Family), died of myocardial infarction at the age of 44.

Medical data proves that populations in high risks of cardiovascular disease are patients with obesity and Triple H. With the improvement of people's living standard, the large group is mightily driving over the cliff of stroke and myocardial infarction, almost 'without hesitation'.

III. Pessimistic Current Situation of China

May 17, 2013, was the seventh 'World Hypertension Day'. In previous media communication meeting, Lisheng Liu, Professor of Fuwai Hospital Chinese Academy of Medical Sciences (President of

World Hypertension League), pointed out that prevalence of hypertension among adults in China reaches up to 33.5% at present. On the basis of estimation, there are over 330 million hypertension patients in China, more than the total population of US. That is to say, there is average one hypertension patient per every three adults. The youth oriented tendency of hypertension is more and more obvious, which is especially worrisome.

According to the report on September 12, 2013, by Bloomberg News, International Diabetes Federation stated that diabetes makes China under great pressure. Last year, China has spent 17 billion US dollars for diabetes.

Now, there are 114 million diabetes patients in China, accounting for 11.6% of Chinese adults. Compared to the estimation of last November by IDF, the actual number exceeds the estimation by 21.6 million patients, almost equal to the total population of Australia. And the prevalence of diabetes in China was only 1% in 1980, 33 years ago.

'It is horrible,' said Daqing Lin, Professor of the University of Hong Kong, 'This is only the start of diabetes epidemic and the most severe situation are yet to come.' Barry Popkin, Professor of the University of North Carolina, thinks: 'This is only the tip of the iceberg. The weight of Chinese younger generation would be much heavier. The prevalence of obesity and diabetes is much higher, and will rise significantly in the future'. In accordance with estimation, there are 500 million people facing the risk of diabetes.

In 1982, a survey on dietary and nutrition found that there were 7% of the population who were overweight. In 1992, a national census on nutrition found that there were 15% of the population who were overweight. In 2002, Chinese Academy of Medical Sciences carried out a most comprehensive research on national diet conditions at that time. The research surveyed 270 thousand people all over the country. Of which, 22.8% Chinese adults were overweight (almost 200 million). General

Administration of Sport publicised the survey result of 43 thousand adults from 10 provinces on August 6, 2013. The survey showed that there are 34.4% overweight people among Chinese people, aged from 20 to 69. For the past 10 years, the average weight gain of Chinese people is almost equal to that of Western for 30 years.

The above data is showed by form as follows,

Statistical Year	Percentage of Overweight
1982	7% Overweight
1992	15% Overweight
2002	22.8% Overweight
2013	34.4% Overweight

On July 26, 2011, the World Bank released a report, titled 'To Create a Healthy and Harmonious Life: Contain China's Chronic Diseases Epidemic', and pointed out that in the next 20 years, the number of patients who would suffer from chronic diseases among Chinese people, aged over 40, will increase by 2-3 times. That is to say, the next 20 years (2010-2030) are the outbreak period of the chronic disease (namely lifestyle disease).

Section Two: Health Risks of Lifestyle Disease

Let's talk specifically about the risks of obesity, Triple H, and cardiovascular disease to personal health.

I. Risks of Obesity

Compared to the normal people, 'fat people' are more likely to have hypertension, abnormal blood lipid profile and diabetes. So obese patients are not only unhealthy, but also are 'as weak as water'.

Nowadays, the internationally adopted BMI (Body Mass Index) is used to assess human weight status. According to regulations of World

Health Organization: BMI= weight (Kg) ÷ height (m) squared. When BMI is over 24, it is overweight. When BMI is over 28, it is obesity. For example, if one's height is 1.75 meter and his weight is 68 kg, then his BMI=68/1.75/1.75=22.2.

80% of diabetes patients suffer from obesity. Moreover, the longer you suffer from obesity, the greater prevalence of diabetes.

Almost half of obese people suffer from fatty liver (hepatic steatosis).

The incidence of angina and sudden death for obese people is 4 times higher than normal people.

The incidence of having bone and joint diseases is 4 to 5 times of the normal-weight people. Most commonly, the diseases are knee osteoarthritis and femoral head necrosis.

The obese females are more likely to have endometrial cancer and breast cancer after menopause.

The obese males are more likely to have prostate cancer. Also, if they are obese, both men and women are more likely to have colon cancer and rectal cancer.

The more severe obesity you have, the higher risk of having above several cancers.

The obesity has a big influence on the pregnancy women. The medical research shows that there is a 30% less in the chance of conceiving for every 0.1 increase in the ratio of waistline/hipline. So, obesity is a major cause for female infertility. Even if they do successfully conceive, the women who are obese before pregnancy are more likely to have complications of pregnancy, like gestational diabetes, hypertension. In addition, the chance for difficult births due to uterine inertia during labour will increase.

If a caesarean section is carried out, the common complications of obese women are greater blood loss, longer operation time, and greater chance of postoperative infection and so on.

The related research also shows that the women who are obese before pregnancy are more likely to have birth defects than normal-weight people. The probability of foetal neural tube malformation of them is twice as high compared to normal weight people. The probability of foetal spina bifida of them is more than 3 times higher than those of normal weight. The risk of heart malformation of them is 2 times higher than those in the control group. The risk of asgastroschisis and acromphalus of them is over 3 times than those in the control group.

The risks of obesity to children and teenagers cannot be ignored. According to survey, hypertension and hyperlipidaemia prevails among obese children. Also, obesity is the main reason for arteriosclerosis, coronary heart disease and diabetes in adulthood. The research has found that the arteries of quite a few obese teenagers appears early lesions of atherosclerosis, which causes over-thick fat accumulation in cerebral cortex, sulcus to reduce, wrinkles to disappear, so as to limit the development in intelligence.

In addition to the influence on the body, the dangers brought by obesity to the children's psychology can never be ignored. Such as, children always like to make comments on the companions with special shape due to their immaturity. Yet many obese children are very sensitive, which will cause them to generate psychological pressure, reduce self-worth, contact less with others, meaning that it is liable to form the characteristics of isolated, self-contemptuous, even autistic personality. If great attention is not paid, the pathological personality formed in the adolescence is likely to cause pathological life in the future.

II. Hazard of Hypertension

The main complication of hypertension is cerebrovascular disease, especially cerebral haemorrhage. In the 27-month prospective follow-up observational study among 596 elder hypertension patients, the cumulative incidence of cerebrovascular disease is 76.91%.

The research shows that the higher the blood pressure, the higher the incidence rate of complication. Shanghai City carried out a follow-up observation on the relationship between blood pressure and cerebral stroke for 5456 people over 15 years of age. The 9-year–long follow-up observation found that 70% of the cerebrovascular patients suffered from hypertension before. Of which, the relative risk of cerebrovascular disease of patients diagnosed with hypertension is 32 times of person with normal blood.

III. Risks of Hyperlipidaemia

Hyperlipidaemia is like 'blood clotting'. It causes atherosclerosis, which means that the blood vessels are blocked up gradually. The blocked blow vessels result in slower blood flow; if the condition is extremely severe, the blood flow can be chocked off. If hyperlipidaemia happens in the heart, it will cause coronary heart disease. If in the kidney, renal arteriosclerosis and kidney failure can be resulted. If in the lower limbs, it can lead to lower limb necrosis and ulcers etc.

In addition, hyperlipidaemia can cause hypertension, induce gallstones and pancreatitis, aggravate hepatitis, and result in male sexual dysfunction, senile dementia and other diseases. So, hyperlipidaemia is not simply a problem with little higher blood lipids, the danger and risks of it cannot be ignored.

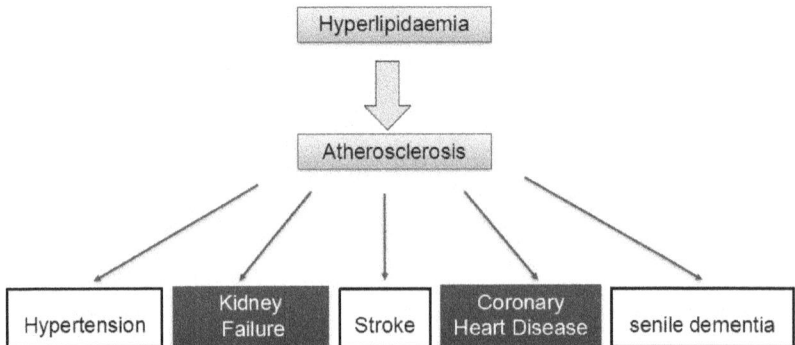

IV. Risks of Diabetes

Diabetes can be divided into Type I and Type II. Of which, Type I Diabetes is also called 'insulin dependent diabetes mellitus'. The patients with this type of diabetes have an absolute lack of insulin, thus they must rely on the insulin treatment. This type of diabetes tends to occur in children and teenagers, while also scattered in other various ages.

Type II Diabetes is also called 'non-insulin dependent diabetes mellitus', or 'adult-onset diabetes'. It is mainly caused by insulin resistance. According to the statistics, over 90% of diabetes patients have Type II diabetes. The diabetes mentioned in this book refers to Type II Diabetes only.

Diabetes will have a direct impact on kidney. The early-stage symptoms are proteinuria and oedema, while kidney failure will happen in the later stage.

Diabetes also threatens our eyes. The hazards to eyeballs include retinopathy and cataract. Diabetes may cause the decreased vision, or blindness under extreme severe conditions.

Cardio-cerebrovascular diseases is the fatal complication of diabetes. It mainly manifests in atherosclerosis of aorta, coronary artery and cerebral artery, endotheliosis of small vessels in whole body, and thickening of capillary walls. The death rate of diabetes patients with cardio-cerebrovascular complication is 3.5 times as high as those without diabetes. This is also a leading cause of death of diabetes.

The risk of the complication to the peripheral vascular is the insufficient blood perfusion of regional tissue. So, the patients are more likely to have local tissue ulceration than average people. The most common are foot ulcers. The clinical manifestations include ache and ulcer of lower limb, while the serious one may cause limb amputation. In this case, amputation is inevitable.

The clinical manifestation of the nervous system from diabetes include: numbness to limbs ending, burning sensation or cold tingle, while in serious case, toss and turn, up all night, and also abnormal sweating, abdominal distension, constipation or diarrhoea, tachycardia or bradycardia, incomplete emptying or urinary incontinence and other symptoms.

Moreover, diabetes is the most common cause for impotence, out of all organic diseases.

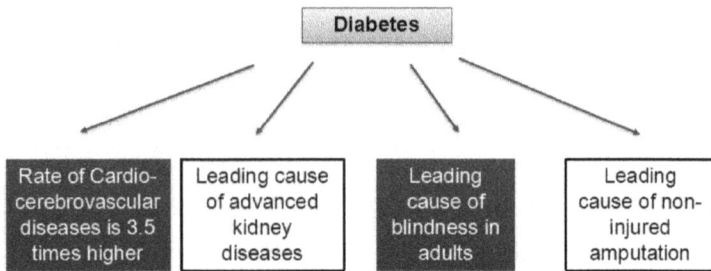

```
                         ┌──────────┐
                         │ Diabetes │
                         └──────────┘
```

Rate of Cardio-cerebrovascular diseases is 3.5 times higher	Leading cause of advanced kidney diseases	Leading cause of blindness in adults	Leading cause of non-injured amputation

V. Risks of Cardio-cerebrovascular Diseases

According to the statistics of Ministry of Health, the first onset age of one third of cardio-cerebrovascular patients in China is under 60. Its morbidity, mortality, disability and recurrence rate are all very high. And it is also easy to induce more complications.

The morbidity of cardio-cerebrovascular diseases reaches up to 13.6%, and has been growing at a rate of 20,000 every day.

Its mortality rate as high as 45%, accounting for 50% of total deaths.

The disability of stroke reaches up to 75%.

The recurrence rate of cardio-cerebrovascular diseases (myocardial infarction and cerebral infarction) within five years at an extremely high rate - 42%.

In addition, there are also a lot of complications of respiratory system, digestive system and urinary system, which are triggered by cardio-cerebrovascular accidents.

Section Three: Societal Risks of Lifestyle Disease

The above is only the risks of lifestyle disease to health of an individual. Let's talk about the risks to society next.

I. Devour Social Wealth

The difference between lifestyle disease and natural disasters lies in the long course of disease, long treatment, and patients are likely to gain more complications during the course. So, it devours plenty of social wealth.

Take diabetes for example, according to the statistics shown in the article published in the New England Journal of Medicine, the direct medical spending for diabetes accounts for 13% of total health expenditure in China, as high as 17.34 billion RMB. The medical service used by diabetes patients is three to four times of non-diabetics (including the great increase in the number of both hospitalisation and outpatient clinics). In the future 10 to 20 years, the figures will rise even higher and more rapidly.

The medical expenses for the patients with over 10-year course of disease are 460% high than those with one-year to two-year course. The medical expenses for diabetes patients are nine times of those non-diabetes persons with same age and same sex. According to the assessment of International Diabetes Federation, if all Chinese diabetes patients accept the treatment funded by the government regularly, then more than half of the annual Chinese medial budgets may be expended on the disease.

More than 300 million patients with Triple H need repeated medication and treatment during the period living with diseases, this may continue for 10 to 30 years, which occupies a lot of medical resource. To some extent, it can be said that the scarce resources are the reasons for the difficulty of getting medical service for everyone.

The expense for lifestyle disease in early stage is not much. However, if it is be controlled in time, it will affect heart and cerebral vessels in later stage. Then the chronic disease will transform into acute disease. The emergency medical expense for it at the onset of disease will become extremely great, and will keep on rising. The China Cardiovascular Disease Report in 2012 published on the China Heart Conference (CHC), held in September 2013 in Beijing, pointed out that general expense for patients with three great cardiovascular diseases - acute myocardial infarction, intracranial haemorrhage and cerebral infarction, in China was more than RMB 46 billion in 2011. Of which, the highest general expense was cerebral infarction, as high as RMB 27.296 billion; intracranial haemorrhage, RMB 14.156 billion; acute myocardial infarction up to RMB 4.987 billion. After adjusting for price changes (i.e. inflation), the total cost has grown at an average annual rate of 25% since 2004, that is double the amount every about three years, which is far above the level that normal person can bear. What a horrific figure!

China is a developing country. We establish technology superpower with the great Chinese Dream of national rejuvenation, so we need to devote a lot of expenditure to set up innovation-oriented society. Yet, our government budget for basic education for all citizens is insufficient. The education in poor rural area is much worse. At the same time, we need to invest a lot of money to pollution control due to our worsening environment. Nevertheless, the limited wealth created by us is devoured mercilessly by the 'black hole' of lifestyle disease.

From the evidence, it can be seen that it is a kind of economy, a type of investment, a responsibility for personal health and a support for development of the nation, to gain health lifestyle and have a healthy body.

II. Lower Quality of Citizens

The statement of which lifestyle disease may lower national quality is not claimed without proper considerations. The findings of a medical sampling, published by Shenyang Physical Examination Centre, shows that there are 50.24% of civil servants getting obesity, while the rate of obese entrepreneurs is up to 64.64%. Civil servants and entrepreneurs are the political elites and economic elites of the whole country respectively, they control the primary power and wealth of the society. Elites are facing more serious impedes from lifestyle disease, which results in the decline of national overall competitiveness.

80% of the obesity of children and adolescents will become adult 'fat people'. China will be strong if the young is strong. The increasingly serious obesity of children and adolescents has lowered physical quality of a generation without a doubt. The decline in learning ability caused by IQ drop is also inevitable.

Before that, the obesity of pregnant women is proved to lower the quality of infants, and increase prevalence rate of various disease. Namely, the obesity of previous generation will definitely result in the decline of overall quality of next generation. Then our next generation will fall behind at the starting line when they are just born.

The negative effects of lifestyle disease on citizen quality are extensive and unprecedented. In the modern history, except for the opium, there is nothing that can weaken a nation as much as the lifestyle disease. One person living with lifestyle disease is an individual and a family tragedy. A generation suffering from lifestyle disease is a tragedy of the nation. If we do not take effective actions to solve this problem, the tragedy is unavoidable. There is absolutely no exaggerations in this claim.

III. Threaten Social Security

A lot of obese patients need to consume more food, which is the most important and basic resource of a country. Food safety is an overall significant strategic issue which not only concerns the survival of people, but also the national economic development, social stability and nation independence in China.

We support 22% of population with 9% cultivated land. The land has now been overwhelmed and overdrawn severely. The soil problems, ecological environment problems and security issues of agricultural products caused by the excessive use of chemical pesticides have slowly taken place. The irreversible urbanisation in the future 20 years will aggravate the tension of cultivated land. Although the food output in China has been rising for nine consecutive years, the average increase in the recent five years (2008-2012) was only 3.28%. The food security situation is still difficult. The times of increasing food product through yielding solely may be difficult to continue.

British Daily Mail quoted a research report on June 18, 2016, saying that the heavier the individual weight is, the more energy they need. The reason for it is that movement of bodies requires energy. Even if the bodies are still, the heavier one will consume relatively more energy than the normal-weight one. The report pointed out that the increase in food demand of the world caused by overweight population was equal to the food demand of one billion people. So, it is not the quantity of the population, but weight of the population, which is the main threat to food security. The enlightenment drawn from the research is that the means of solving lifestyle disease is critical to the solution of national food security.

The lifestyle disease would not only become the burden of family, but even a heavy burden on the country. The lifestyle disease patients always retire early due to the disease, and it is necessary to have someone to replace the vacancy, which increases the production costs. At the same time, people tend to develop these diseases at a younger age, which would worsen the already significant shortage in labour with no doubts.

Professor Popkin from University of North Carolina emphasised that if the trend of obesity in China is not effectively controlled, the obesity will slow down its economic growth rate in the future five to ten years. GDP increase at a medium-to-high speed has important strategic significance to keep the social stability in China. The long-term yet outstanding damage to human resource caused by lifestyle disease will hold back the rapid growth of Chinese economy, which will threaten the development and stability of the country.

Chapter Two: How Is Lifestyle Disease Developed

Section One: Poor Lifestyle Is the Main Cause for the Disease

I. The Blood, Sweat, and Tears behind 'Popeye'

If we want to control and treat the disease, we must first know the cause of the disease.

I believe that you must have some memories of 'Popeye' as you company your children to watch cartoons sometimes. Popeye has infinite strength when he eats spinach, then any difficult tasks will become easy for him, yet there is a tragic history hidden behind the vivid story.

For about 500 years, from 15th century to 20th century, the sailors on long sea voyages faced the risk of deaths all the time. Because there was a disease called 'scurvy', which took the lives of hundreds of thousands of sailors successively. People always regarded it as an incurable disease due to unclear causes.

Finally, in 1922, people determined the cause of scurvy was vitamin C deficiency. This is because they were unable to eat fresh vegetables due to long sea voyages.

Problems were easily solved after knowing the cause. As long as food which are rich in vitamin C are constantly consumed in an appropriate amount, such lemon juice, fresh fruits and vegetables, the scurvy can be completely prevented and treated. That is obviously where the plot design of Popeye eating spinach comes from.

As can be seen, it is important to know the cause in order to solve problems. As for the prevention and treatment of lifestyle disease, firstly we shall know why people get such disease.

II. Three Poor Lifestyle Habits Which Cause the Sharp Increase in Lifestyle Disease

From long-term research, the medical experts and pathologists have found that the main cause for the outbreak of lifestyle disease is the unhealthy lifestyle. Of which three points are especially noticeable, namely 'eating too much', 'eating wrongly',

And 'lack of exercise'. Of which, the most important cause is 'eating too much'.

In 2004, UK Times quoted a scientific conclusion, 'Overeating is much worse to health than lifelong smoking and drinking.' An experiment consisting of a group of laboratory rats eat more than enough for every meal, while the other groups of laboratory rats eat till only 70% to 80% full, had supported this statement. The results showed that average lifetime of the rats that eat too much had reduced by 40%.

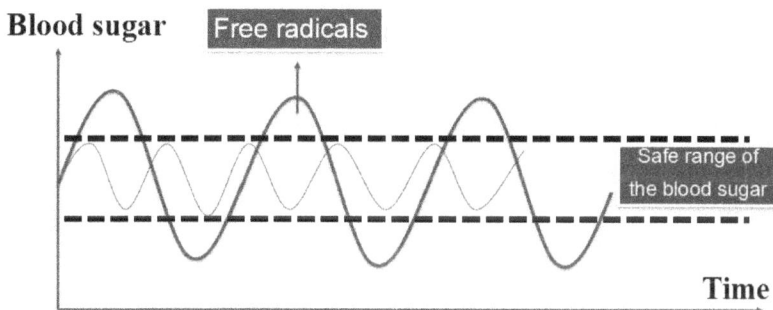

Figure One: Eating Too Much

What exactly is wrong with eating too much?

Overeating may increase the burden on metabolism. Let's look at the Figure One. The two straight, horizontal dotted lines represent the relatively small and safe range the blood sugar should fluctuate in. Three large peaks mean that blood sugar may rise after every meal (three meals a day).

We all know that the function of human pancreas is to secrete insulin which lowers the blood sugar levels. Overeating will cause the blood sugar to rise too much, which forces pancreas to overload and accelerate insulin secretion. It will result in overdrawing and failure of pancreas.

The smaller wavy lines between two dotted lines represent multiple meals with small amount of food for each, which is 70% to 80% full for dinner, and addition of appropriate snacks. In this way, blood sugar fluctuation and load of pancreas are smaller, the regulatory function of blood sugar is not as likely to decline.

In addition, too high impacts of blood sugar will produce plenty of endogenous free radicals. Free radicals firstly may oxidize the weakest capillary endothelium, which will result in inflammation and thickening of blood capillary. We will analyse this phenomenon later in greater details.

For 'eating wrongly', it is the actual most important cause for the lifestyle disease. We will have a special discussion on it in the next chapter.

We will first talk about two issues caused by lack of exercise.

One is that decline in binding power of insulin receptors of membranes. There is a door for in and out of blood sugar on the edge of the membrane, called insulin receptor. When the binding power of receptor declines, it can be simply thought as the door is rusty and cannot be opened. So, the blood sugar will have troubles as it enters the cell. The research shows that aerobic exercise may reverse the decline in binding power of insulin receptors of myocardial membranes.

Two is the depletion in number of mitochondria in cells. The mitochondrion is a place for energy metabolism. The blood sugar will complete burning after it enters the mitochondrion. A profound study has found that the number of mitochondria in human cells may decline with aging. When lack of exercise, the decline will be accelerated, the speed of metabolism will decrease. A study shows that the aerobic exercise will increase the number of mitochondria.

Section Two 'Eating Wrongly' is the Key Risk Factor

The so-called 'Eating Wrongly' mainly refers to eating wrong staple food, which means that too much of refined grains are consumed, or disproportionate ratio between coarse and refined grains. This is the main cause for obesity and Triple H.

I. Healthy Eating Pyramid by Harvard University

Figure Two is 'Healthy Eating Pyramid by Harvard University' published by U.S. Department of Agriculture in 2005. Healthy Eating Pyramid by Harvard University is a significant scientific summary by Harvard University, Yale University and more than ten other universities, which took ten years, costed 100 million US Dollars and had follow-up surveys on dietary structure of about 0.1 million people. The food pyramid is adopted as the national standard by U.S. Department of Agriculture as the guide to dietary structure of the public. We should eat more food that are closer to the pyramid's base and less food closer to pyramid's tip.

Let's focus on the staple food: located at the tip are 'white rice, refined noodle, potatoes, sweetener', with the reminder of 'eating less'. At the base is the 'whole grains', with reminder of '(to eat in) each meal'. Namely the Healthy Eating Pyramid by Harvard University suggests us to base our staple food on coarse grains. Yet in fact, most of us consume refined grains as staple food.

The refined grain is the remaining part of whole grain after the removal of the bran. Its major ingredient is starch, which in in fact sugar. The bran is rich in vitamin, mineral and fibre. It is a shame to waste all of them. So, the refined grain only provides calories, but no traces of elements which help to burn the calories. It will cause unbalanced nutrition if refined grains are consumed frequently, which will exacerbate the unbalance of metabolism, which finally triggers metabolic diseases.

THE HEALTHY EATING PYRAMID

Department of Nutrition, Harvard School of Public Health

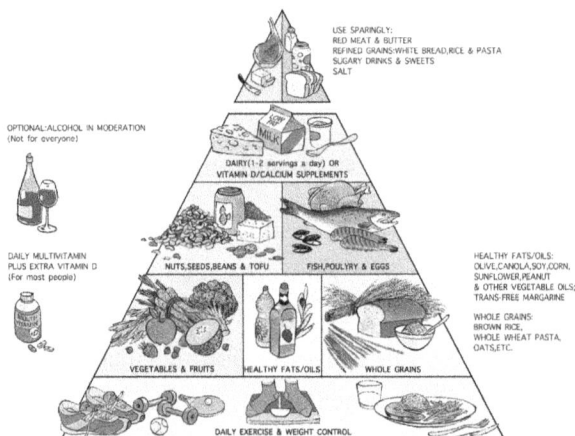

Figure Two: Healthy Eating Pyramid by Harvard University

II. Rule of 20 Years by Thomas L. Cleave

The internationally recognized 'Rule of 20 Years' points out that: if people in a country or a district changed their staple food into refined carbohydrate, the diabetes and cardiovascular disease will appear within 20 years; and these diseases will spread within 40 years. Thomas L. Cleave is a doctor for the UK Royal Navy. His Rule of 20 Years was certified in Iceland, Israel, Saudi Arabia, India, Japan, Mexico and many other countries. Now China is verifying the principle.

Many people mistakenly believe that abundant fish and meat are the main cause for obesity and Triple H. Yet middle and old aged women rarely eat lavish meals and they still are generally fat. Also, patients of fatty liver and Triple H can be found everywhere. Why? The answer is simple: eating too much of refined grains.

III. Glycaemic Index (GI)

Why are refined grains so dangerous? Doctor David J. Jenkins, from University of Toronto, has put forward the well-known concept of 'Glycaemic Index (GI)' in 1981, which shocked the medical field. It brings people's knowledge about carbohydrate to a whole new level.

Before 1981, people classified carbohydrate simple carbohydrate and complex carbohydrate using early 20th century knowledge. Yet after the introduction to the theory of GI, people can understand how carbohydrate works in human body to a deeper level.

'Journal of American Medical Association' issued an analysis review on 311 researches regarding GI on August 5th, 2002. This suggested that the medical field accepted the concept of GI more and more.

The research by Professor Walter C. Willett, a member of American Academy of Sciences and Dean of Nutrition Department of Harvard University, shows that eating food with high GI will cause the increase of blood sugar and insulin level, which will cause hypertension, cholesterol and high level of triglyceride and other factors which may trigger heart disease.

GI is an effective index to weigh the postprandial glycaemic response caused by food. It is a percentage of blood sugar increase caused by 50g carbohydrate food and 50g glucoses within a certain time (usually two hours). It is a relative numerical value which reflects the speed and capacity of increasing blood sugar caused by food and glucoses. The GI of glucoses is usually set as 100, as shown in Figure Three. The food with high GI may cause the rapid increase of postprandial blood sugar and brings a serious impact on blood sugar, and food with low GI will slowly increase blood sugar and brings a gentle burden on blood sugar.

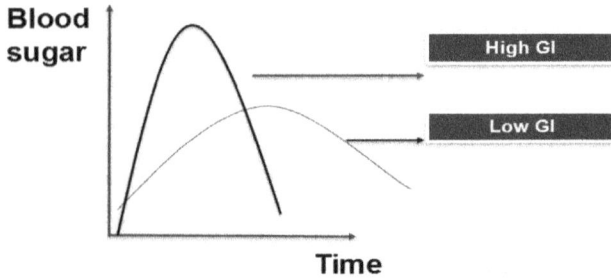

Figure Three: Glycaemic Index (GI)

Generally speaking, the food with GI≥75 is high GI. It is digested rapidly after into the stomach, with high absorption rate and rapid glucose release. The peak value is high after the glucose goes into the blood. On the other hand, the food with GI < 55 is low GI. It will stay in the stomach for a longer time, with lower absorption rate and slower glucose release. It can prevent postprandial high blood sugar.

The food with GI between 51 and 75 is mid GI, as shown in Figure Four. GI of brown rice is 56, corn 55, rice 84, white steamed bread 88, white bread 88, white sugar 83.8. GI of white sugar is lower than that of rice and steamed bread. This may not be what is normally expected by the majority of people.

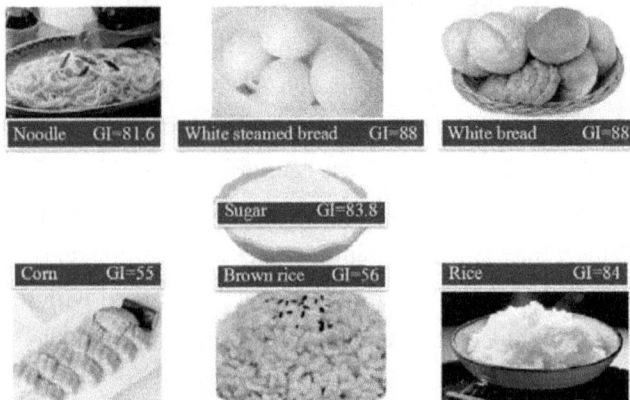

Figure Four: GI of Common Staple Food

In summary, the more processed the carbohydrates are, the higher the GI. The GI of rice and white bread are equivalent to sugar. Having refined grains every meal will heavily push up postprandial blood sugar, just like having sugar each meal and increase the burden of the pancreas. It can be seen that it is not too much sugar, but too much refined grains which cause so common diabetes.

IV. Carbohydrate Addiction

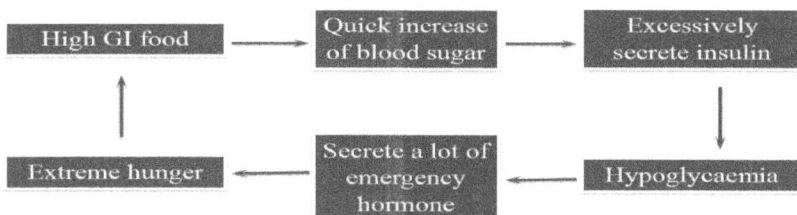

Figure Five: Eating Wrongly -- Carbohydrate Addiction

Long-term intake of high GI food will lead to 'carbohydrate addiction'. The diet survey shows that 85% of food we intake every day is high GI. For example, rice porridge, white steamed bread, steamed stuffed bun and deep-fried dough sticks we usually eat for breakfast, are all high GI food.

As shown in Figure Five, intake of one meal of 'high GI food' will cause 'quick increase of blood sugar' after the meal. Then pancreas will 'excessively secrete insulin' to lower blood sugar, which will cause 'hypoglycemia'. Hypoglycemia brings dizziness, palpitation, limbs atony, lack of strength, sweating, 'black out' episode etc. The human body will 'secrete a lot of emergency hormone', which brings 'extreme hunger', which will make people to seek for food.

At lunchtime, the rice or noodles we have are again 'high GI food', then still 'quick increase of blood sugar' after meal, then pancreas will 'excessively secrete insulin' to cause 'hypoglycemia', 'secrete a lot of emergency hormone', and bring 'extreme hunger'. So the vicious circle is formed.

The extreme hunger brought by high GI food is more likely to cause overeating. That is to say, eating wrongly can lead to eating too much more easily. Eating too much and eating wrongly will drive the vicious circle together to cause 'carbohydrate addiction'. The main performance is craving for staple food. That is to say, no matter how much dishes we got in a meal, we will feel hungry if there are no carbohydrates.

The high sugar level after eating keeps stimulates the organs to secret insulin in order to control blood sugar. However, this will lead to the deaths of many pancreatic islets, and decrease in our ability to control sugar level on our own.

What is more, the serious impact on postprandial sugar blood will produce a large number of endogenous free radicals to accelerate aging and quicken the formation of metabolic disturbance. There will be specific discussion for this concept later.

Chapter Three: Fight between Two Medical Models
(Selective reading for patients, compulsory reading for practitioners)

Facing the growing population with lifestyle disease and its harm, the traditional biomedical model is rather helpless.

The medical model, also called medical pattern, is the general principal and starting point followed when people consider and research medical problems, and the philosophy that people know health and disease, including concept of health, concept of disease, concept of diagnose, concept of treatment etc. The traditional 'biomedical model' is the summary to the mainstream medicine in the 19th and 20th century

The biomedical pattern regards human as a biologic organism, and has an intensive study on human body based on biological science. It looks for measurable form or chemical change in human organs, tissues, cells or biological macromolecules, and then confirms biological or physicochemical reasons, finally finds the therapeutic method.

Because the traditional biomedical pattern is rather powerless for the lifestyle disease, we put forward another new treating method – 'Wisdom Model of Behavioural Health'. Let's compare it with the traditional method. Of course, it does not mean to overwhelm and oppose against biomedical pattern. In fact, these two methods may work together.

Section One: Rethink Old Medical Thinking - 'Biomedical Model'

I. Advantages of Biomedical Model

The scientific reasoning supporting biomedical model is 'reductionism'. So-called 'reduction' is thought in general that a realm of phenomenon can be concluded to a lower or deeper realm of phenomenon for it to be understood. The core ideology of reductionism is that the world is made up of individuals. The reductionism focuses on making difficult things simple, and breaking up the whole into parts. The modern physics attributes the existence of the world to fundamental particles and their interactions with 'reduction'. The biologists explain the complex phenomena of all animals and plants by cells and devote themselves to shedding light on all mysteries of vital complexity by the research of molecular level.

From the establishment of cell theory of three discoveries of natural science in the 19th century till now, biomedicine developed significantly. People's thorough understanding to cells, bacteria, viruses and macro human structure and function in micro fields, as well as a serious of medical achievements built accordingly, which makes biomedical model become mature gradually.

The main achievements of biomedical pattern are embodied in two aspects:

Detection method: invention of various kinds of physical examination devices and all kinds of laboratory test methods;

Treatment method: invention of antibiotics and vaccines in the medicine; solve the issues of pain, infection and loss of blood by anaesthesia, sterilization and blood transfusion in the surgery.

The biomedical model made an ever-lasting contribution to human health in the last century. Under the guidance of biomedical model, humans basically have solved the infectious diseases, which had threatened human health for thousands of years. The spectrum of disease has undergone a fundamental change, and the average life expectancy has been raised greatly.

II. Limitations of Biomedical Model

The biomedical model can be said to consider the disease only but no patients. It largely ignores the individual characteristics, psychological factor of patients and the adaptation of individual to society and natural environment. In the field of fatal infectious diseases and surgeries, the biomedical model has got a great success, which makes people habitually apply the mechanical thinking to discuss and research the cause and treatment of other diseases. For cancer, diabetes, hypertension and some other complex chronic diseases, people also seek for the static and direct relation between these diseases and some specific proteins and genes. They hope to control the function of specific protein or the expression of specific genes to achieve the goal of treatment and prevention.

The current popular researches, like targeted therapy, drug design and search for cause of genome-wide, are all the extension and expansion of the same thinking and methodology. Most of the researches are very strict and no doubt quite valuable. Yet, the attempts which apply research results to the clinic to prevent and treat diseases are often frustrating.

Many people are optimistic that this is only due to the limits of technology. We are unable to discuss the cell physiology in the molecular level more clearly. Once the technology is good enough, people may find specific pathogenesis of complex diseases by direct or digital biological research pattern, and then target to have an intervention treatment. The thinking cannot be called unreasonable. However, in the present, when the life science has got so broad and deep achievements, and human has got our own blueprint of life — genomes, the biomedical model seemingly has no capacity to make full use of these achievements to provide better and more effective medical service for people.

The investment of medical research and drug development is greater and greater, but the output is smaller and smaller. The high expense for research and development are all passed to general patients, which make the cost of outpatient visits higher and higher, and the quality improvement in medical service lags far behind the rise of price.

III. To Solve a Problem, the Correct Tool Must Be Used

In the contemporary society, the diseases caused by biological factors (like infectious disease) have declined, but the diseases caused by social factors (like lifestyle disease) have become prominent. At the end of 20th century, and the beginning of 21st century, human has ushered in lifestyle disease. Facing new problems, the biomedical model has suffered a major setback and increasingly felt overwhelmed.

For example: there is a yard which needs to be cleaned up, with the ground covered with leaves and strewn with some stones. The traditional biomedical model is like a broom. It is really good to sweep the fallen leaves, but rather powerless to sweep the stones. However, the inertia makes us to sweep constantly, if one time is not okay, then try to sweep for more times; if this broom is not okay, then change the brooms. It causes the overuse of the broom, but cannot get a good effect. The more sweeping, the more frustrated people feel. At this moment, if we change to another way of thinking, and add a 'tool', the problem will be solved.

Yes, indeed. Obesity, Triple H etc. are like those stones. Taking diabetes, hypertension as example, the advantages and limitations of the biomedical model are very obvious. The alternative medicines, like anti-diabetic drugs and hypertensive drugs, are a great progress of human medicine. The effective control on blood sugar and blood pressure brings down the high mortality rate caused by acute attack and largely extend the disease-carrying survival time. Its contributions cannot go unnoticed, but the intrinsic limitations of drugs alternative therapy are exposed more and more apparently. For example:

1. It can only control, but not cure

Alternative agents have no significant help in the recovery of body's own function. The essence of substitution is that the body originally has hypotension and hypoglycemic functions, now the functions weaken, result in the elevation of blood sugar and blood pressure, so drugs replace the original functions of body. That is to say, the alternative therapy does commit itself to recover body function. So it certainly has no significant help in the disease rehabilitation.

2. Drug dependence, liver and kidney damage

Drug alternative will lead to the dependence. Just like the son does not do homework and father replace him to do it. The result is that the more replacement, the more dependent the son is on his father. Long-term substitution will cause the constant weakening of the body's functions. So, if the patient stopped using drugs after a period of time, the condition would be worsened. On the other hand, taking medication all the year around will aggravate the liver and kidney damages and increase the risk of liver cirrhosis and renal failure with more and more dosage.

3. Accelerate the formation of complication

Taking type II diabetes as an example, the patients themselves can produce insulin, it's just the decrease of activity or can be said that the insulin is not sensitive, so it leads to somewhat higher blood sugar. Insulin injections are unable to improve the activity of insulin. They are just to increase the insulin concentration in the blood. Although the blood sugar is declined to the normal range, at the cost of causing 'hyperinsulinemia', which will further accelerate clotting of blood platelet. It is more likely to form hardening of arteries, and accelerate the formation of cerebral infarction and myocardial infarction. So, although the blood sugar levels of patients are controlled within the normal range, most of them still die of complications, like stroke and myocardial infarction, earlier than the normal.

Section Two: Put Forward New Medical Thinking – 'Wisdom Model of Behavioural Health'

Because the traditional biomedical model has no effects on the lifestyle diseases well as the intrinsic requirement of lifestyle disease, the Team of Doctor Lu has put forward a new 'Wisdom Model of Behavioural Health'.

The 'behavioural health' refers to the correct lifestyle; 'wisdom' has two meanings: one is cell wisdom – cell wisdom is inherent and has a powerful capability for self-healing; another one is wisdom of human – improve health awareness, know and comply with objective patterns.

In principle, the 'Wisdom Model of Behavioural Health' both pays attention to the natural property of human, and focuses on the social property of human. In practice, it develops 'reductionism' and 'holism' simultaneously. On the basis of comprehensively and profoundly understanding of the mechanism of lifestyle disease, the model puts forward clear guiding principles for practice.

I. Balance the Importance between Natural Property and Social Property

The natural property of human refers to the physical characteristics and biological characteristics, such as the need for food and drinks, the instinct of defence, the wants for sexual interactions etc. The social property means the relationship properties formed and developed among people on the basis of social practice, for example, the dependency of human symbiotic relationship, social interactions (physically, mentally and emotionally) in the interpersonal relationships, morality and ethics, cooperation in the producing activity etc.

The lifestyle disease is not only a problem derived from human itself, but also a problem of socialization. So we can only comprehensively and correctly know the essential of lifestyle disease by considering both the natural property and social property.

On the one hand, consider natural properties of human:

• Understand the human instinct better in virtue of the deep knowledge of cells from biomedicine;

• Create conditions to better exercise human instinct through the research achievement of nutrition and exercise science;

• Carry out quantitative research and evaluation on the health condition, and guide the process of improvement by various kinds of physiochemical indexes for physical examination;

• Ensure the stability of metabolic index with the help of the control of drugs, in order to restore and re-establish a stable physiological environment for a cell by instincts.

On the other hand, consider the social properties of human:

• Evaluate carefully the impacts of food industrialization and agricultural modernization on the dietary pattern and quality of modern human, and establish corresponding countermeasure for nutritional enhancement;

• Give full consideration to the change of working nature of the modern people, like the impacts of reduction of physical labour and increase of mental labour on human metabolism, and put forward simple exercise programs for specific working pace and working environment.

• Respond actively to the impacts of social interaction with a richer variety of forms, and various dinners and banquets etc. on the dietary patterns of the modern. Not only provide preventive strategies, but also provide remedial action afterwards.

• Give proper consideration to impacts of family culture on individual dietary habits, and the positive and negative roles of family culture plays in the process of establishing new lifestyle, hence take the family into consideration when managing, rather than merely considering the individuals;

• In particular, consider human's mental properties (part of social properties), including the change in the understanding of health concepts, renewal of health knowledge, improvement of health consciousness etc. and make education be carried out to the whole process of health intervention.

II. Develop 'Reductionism' and 'Holism' Simultaneously

According to 'reductionism', the complex system can be explained by the behaviours and its interactions of each part. The reductionism method is the most basic way of natural science research up until now. People tend to observe the behaviours and nature of elements composing of the system through a static and isolated viewpoint. Then the description of the whole system is formed by 'assemble' these properties.

For example, in order to inspect life, we firstly investigate the functions and effects of each part, like the nervous system, digestive system and immune system. When inspecting the systems, we need to know every single organ which is included in each system. If we want to know about organs, we should inspect tissues, at the end, we need to investigate cells, protein, genetic materials, molecules, atoms etc. The well-developed modern science shows that the reductionism is a relatively reasonable research technique. It is certainly worthwhile to seek for and study the most basic component of substance.

In contrast to 'reductionism', 'holism' believes that there are limits to break the system into each component; the highly complex system is usually especially interconnected, it doesn't work to investigate by the practice. So, it is better to investigate things by the viewpoint of holism systematic theory.

For inspecting a complex piece of machinery, the reductionists may immediately pick up a screwdriver and a wrench to break it into thousands or tens of thousands of parts, and inspect them individually. It takes a long time and may not achieve the desired result. The holists will not do this; they will adopt much easier ways. They do not break the machinery into parts, but try to start it, input some directive operation, observe its response and establish the relationship between input and output. Then the functions of the whole machinery can be understood.

Holism is basically functionalism. What holists try to know is overall functionality. They don't burden themselves with how the system functions. It can simplify the problem, but may also lose some important information.

It is necessary to combine reductionism with holism to solve lifestyle disease. The two methods are not better than each other in any way, but they are highly complementary. The strength of reductionism lies in the inspection to the parts and micro. The strength of reductionism lies in the grasp of the whole and macro. The reductionism is good at explaining the whole by parts, and the holism explaining the parts by the whole.

The highly complexity of human body decides the high degree of limitations of using solely one method out of the two. If we do not reduce to the level of cell to a single molecule, we will not understand the refined structure of the part, and our knowledge of the entirety is only intuitive, general and lack of science. If there is no holistic viewpoint, our knowledge to human body is only piecemeal. We will fail to have an overall grasp of things and solve the problem. So, we need to develop 'reductionism' and 'holism' simultaneously.

On the one hand, we should apply the existing experience and technology of reductionism. Specifically, make full use of the cell theory of modern medicine, modern nutrition, biochemical engineering and other techniques (we will discuss them one by one later); on the other hand, apply the concept and thinking of holism. It is concretely expressed as the overall grasp of three levels.

1. Whole human body

It is not confined to one certain organ or one certain clinical index, but looks at the whole body. Although it still pays attention to the part, it adjusts the part while based on the whole. Human body is a complex system of ruling without intervention. Nowadays science has not yet fully figured out all of the secrets of the human body. Yet we can follow the nature of the body, take care of the human instinct, give full play to the system function of body, and improve the part better based on full adjustment.

2. Body and mind

Not only pay attention to the body conditioning, but also pay more attention to the construction of psychology, including change of health concept, improvement of health consciousness, building of health confidence, and development of self-controlling ability etc. All these should be present throughout the education of health interventions.

3. Human and nature

The oriental medicine always emphasizes that 'nature and man in one' and advocates to set up harmony of human and nature. But it is worth noting that nature today is different from what it was a thousand years ago. Human activities have profoundly changed the nature, including air, water, soil and food. The social properties of human have determined that human is not able to escape from society and return to nature, but human needs to live in the modern civilization to adapt the changing nature. Specifically, it is necessary to adapt changes from two aspects:

One is environmental pollution: reduce the level of pollution by all kinds of methods, meanwhile intensify self-purification function of the human body.

The other one is the decline of food quality: global population is unprecedented. It has reached seven billion in 2011, and will reach 9.6 billion in 2050. The huge demand for food has resulted in agricultural modernization. Largely using of fertilizer has caused soil overdraft, and the use of starter and ripening agent has shortened crop grooving season. The agricultural modernization has brought decline of food quality while increasing food supply. Although the modern society still establishes important connection with the nature by food, but the necessary nutrition obtained is relatively insufficient. Especially the general lack of trace elements has exacerbated the nutritional imbalance of the modern society, leading to further imbalanced metabolism. So, nutrient enrichment has become necessary method to maintain health for the modern.

III. Three Guiding Principles in Practice

There are three guiding principles in the practice of 'Wisdom Model of Behavioural Health', namely 'patients first, physicians next', 'education first, medical treatment next', and 'instinct first, science and technology next'. They are discussed in turn as follows:

1. Patient first, physician next

Many people believe that fitness level has much to do with medical care. But ultimately, being healthy relies more on ourselves. Among the factors which influence lifespan, published by World Health Organization, the genetic inheritance accounts for 15%, social and natural environment 17%, and medical care 8% and personal lifestyle 60%. That is to say, all medical treatment factors, including professionals, hospitals, medicine, physician examinations, surgeries etc. accumulate to only be accounted as 8%. While our personal factors account for as much as 60%. Its influence is equivalent to 7.5 times as much as the sum of all medical treatment factors.

Data shows that the average lifespan of Chinese emperors in different dynasties was only 42 years old. Being the emperors, they possessed the most high-end medical resources, but they did not live for a long time. It fully showed that any drug or high-skilled doctor cannot replace a healthy lifestyle. The ultimate path to health and longevity is self-salvation.

Nowadays, whether in the mother country or abroad; whether Traditional Chinese Medicine or Western Medicine; also whether 'mainstream medicine', or 'non-mainstream medicine', patients are usually regarded as the subject who passively accepts treatment. The treatment methods like medicine and surgeries, which are set up mainly by doctors, really play a major role in the diseases caused by trauma, bacteria and viruses etc.

However, for lifestyle disease, the main prescription made by physicians is not drug prescription, but behaviour prescription. The physicians make a prescription for the patients to implement it. The degree of knowledge and implementation of patients to the prescriptions have become the main factors to influence rehabilitation results.

So, the key to Wisdom Model of Behavioural Health is to mainly focus on the patients. The doctors are only allies.

2. Education first, medical treatment next

The fundamental way to solve lifestyle disease is training, setting up healthy behaviour pattern and forming lifelong habit. Patients should have abundant health awareness to set up a healthy behaviour pattern. This mainly relies on education, not treatment. So, we shall place education first, and assist with drugs, surgeries and other medical treatment methods.

Education will make the patient know that why s/he has gotten the lifestyle disease, which behaviour pattern is wrong, why it needs correction and how to correct it. The effective education will make sure the execution of behaviour prescription. Turning new behaviours into living habit and persevere is a fundamental way to keep away from lifestyle disease for life.

This education is a broad education, including thinking education, and behaviour training; including group education, and individual education; including one-way training, as well as two-way interaction.

3. Instinct first, science and technology next

There is no lack of such case in medical practice: after the liver of body is excised by 75%, a new liver can grow within one to two years, and the new liver has the same functions as the original one. What does this mean? Human body has strong self-healing functions.

Human body is born with instincts of metabolizing fats, sugar, uric acid and balancing blood pressure. What we should do is to take care of instincts, recover instincts, create all favourable conditions for them, and get the most out of them.

Technology is far from or even never going to be able to replace human wisdom. The scientific community seeks answers towards technology, but does not seek answers towards our body – the organism that is full of wisdom of the Creator. Human body is a real 'hands-off' intelligence. The father of Western Medicine, Hippocrates, points out that your instinct is your doctor, and the doctor only takes care of your instinct. Our understanding is that the recovery of body mainly relies on the self-healing function of instinct, and all technology can only awaken instincts, assist and strengthen the exercise of instincts.

As for the specific medical plan, we will have special chapters for discussion later. (see Chapter VII)

Chapter Four: Amazing Effects Bring Out Theoretical Innovation

We follow the medical thinking and medical principles advocated by Wisdom Model of Behavioural Health. Through long-term, hard and persevering practice, by repeated adjustment and continuous improvement, we have finally put forward a new theory and developed an effective rehabilitation scheme for lifestyle disease, called 'Cell Comprehensive Revitalisation Program'.

Section One: Amazing Effects, Novel Theories

Before elaborating on the plan, we may firstly look at the actual result brought by implementing the plan. So to speak, in the response to obesity, diabetes, hypertension and other diseases, the effects produced by the plan are unexpected, and incredible. There are a lot of informative and vivid cases attached later in the book. Some examples are given for the sake of explanation here.

I. Amazing Effect is Beyond Question

1. Cases of obesity

As obese patients, most participants can safely lose 5 to 15 kilograms after implementing a short-term plan of one cycle (42 days). During the weight loss, strength, energy, sleep, mood etc. all had been improved significantly, and work and learning efficiency have been obviously improved. The following several cases are relatively notable.

Case one: Hongyu Liu, male, born in 1995, started to implement the plan at the age of 17 (in 2012). In 84 days, he reduced his weight by 53 kilograms (from 146 to 93 kilograms). Meanwhile, his waistline was reduced from 129 to 2.85 centimetres, hipline from 127 to 91 centimetres, and thigh circumference from 82 to 58 centimetres. Fatty liver, myocarditis, arrhythmia and other symptoms all disappeared.

Case two: Xiulan Li, female, in her fifties, lost 35 kilograms within three months.

Case three: Gang Li, male, is 35 years old, with weight 251 kilograms before implementing the plan. He lost 75 kilograms after one cycle of short-term plan. Through a short-term plan of successive three cycles and three-month long-term plan, it reduced to 134 kg (lost 121.5kg). He could not do anything by himself before due to overweight, but he was able to climb up the roof to do construction work after the end of second cycle. He was able to ride a bike after the finish of third cycle (he could not look down at the handlebars when he was riding on the bicycle prior to the treatment).

2. Cases of diabetes:

Excluding the special diabetes patients who had got serious complications in the later period of diabetes, there are 70% to 80% of patients off the pill after implementing one cycle of short-term plan, and other indexes also had been improved. Of which, there were two cases with long course or large dosage:

Case one: Lianyu Zhang, female, 71 years old, had a history of more than 30 years of diabetes. She was injected as many as 103 units of insulin every day before the treatment we provided. Even though she was injected 77 units, and took six anti-diabetic drugs, her fasting glucose still reached up to 14.6 before implementing the plan. After program for 60 days, her fasting glucose was 5.2 with all oral administration stopped and 19 units of insulin every day.

Case two: Jianhua Xue, male, 56 years old, injected insulin pump for 5 years (48 units every day) and took metformin for 10 years before the treatment. After one cycle, all oral administration were stopped, and the insulin pump was removed. Meanwhile he lost over 15 kg and stopped taking lipid-lowering and anti-hypertensive drugs.

Another group data on diabetes getting off the pill in one day Yanda

International Health City held a training camp completely composed of diabetics in 2013. The medical workers in Yanda Hospital took tests of fasting blood glucose for three times every day. There were 38 persons participating in the plan. Of which, 3 people did not implement the plan according to requirements, which were invalid data. There were five people among the other 35 persons who stopped taking medicines in one day, with drug withdrawal rate 14.3%. The concept of drug withdrawal does not mean recovery in one day, rather, it suggests that if the fasting blood glucose in the next morning is lower than 6.1, then patients cannot take medicine anymore, or hypoglycemic will be developed. As for further stabilizing, more time is needed.

3. Cases of hypertension

Excluding the group who had experienced cerebral haemorrhage and had done a heart bypass operation before the treatment, the drug withdrawal rate after one cycle reached up to 70% - 80%, with the improvement of other indexes. There were several cases with severe problems which were later cured.

Case one: Jiange Wang, male, 52 years old, had hypertension for 18 years, and a 15-year drug-taking history. He halved anti-hypertensive drugs after 7 days, and stopped taking the medicine after 15 days after implementing the plan. Meanwhile he lost 12.5 kg, his blood sugar returned to normal and 22-year of sleep disorders was cured.

Case two: Fang Hou, female, 74 years old, had hypertension for over 40 years. She could not control blood pressure within the normal scope even with two and a half anti-hypertensives tablets every day. After one cycle of the treatment, she only takes half a tablet each day, with blood pressure of 120/70.

Case three: Mr. Yuan, male, was 76 years old. The first cerebral infarction happened at the age of 38, and respectively one time at the age of 42 and 45. With hypertension accompanied with diabetes and hyperlipidaemia, he took five to eight different types of medicine every day. He stopped all medicines after one cycle, and his blood pressure and blood sugar restored to normal. The frequency of angina was reduced from 10-12 times every day to once every two to three days.

II. Proposal of New Theory and New Model

The magical effect made our team excited. We had tried to explain it with various kinds of theories, but we had found that the theories did not explain the whole phenomenon fully. We had successively tried heat balance theory, enzyme technology, low-carbs concept, ketogenic technology and meridian theory, but all these had obvious limitation.

On the one hand, we were unable to clearly explain that why the speed of improvement was so quick, and the effect was so noticeable; on the other hand, why the problems, which appeared other methods, did not appear in our results, like malnutrition, cutis laxa, decrease in muscle mass, bone mineral density descending, joint injury, lesions of liver and kidney, constipation, diarrhoea etc.

We were unable to explain it in theory, but we were certain about the effects of the treatment. So, in addition to be amazed at the human instinct, we started to think whether there exists a certain undiscovered physiological mechanism or we should put forward new ideas to explain the phenomenon. At last, we had put forward the theory of 'energy path' and 'energy conversion'.

In practice, we had further found that the patients (who have been treated by us) have changed not only in the bodies, but also in behaviours. Many people had managed to maintain the weight and avoid relapses of Triple H for a long term thanks to a new lifestyle. Nevertheless, these results still could not be explained fully by the theory of 'energy path' and 'energy conversion'. So, we started to think about a medical model. We arrived at the new model from human physiological, psychology and behaviour perspectives, even from social and environmental perspectives. We finally summarized the medical thinking and practice principles, which have guided us to successful practice for many years, including concept of instinct, holistic view, people oriented, education cantered etc. as a new medical model. That's how the 'Wisdom Model of Behavioural Health' was put forward

The one-stop solution has experienced two phases of evolution in the long-term practice: pursue of more efficiency and simplicity. The previous state is mainly addition: trying as many methods which are good for improving lifestyle disease as possible; the later stage is subtraction: drawing a clear distinction between the primary and the secondary, giving up secondary methods, simplifying main methods as much as possible, even appropriately exchanging effect for simplicity. Finally, we arrived at 'Cell Comprehensive Revitalisation Program'.

The lifestyle disease can be cured. Medicines can be stopped for diabetes and hypertension. It is also feasible to solve lifestyle disease with a different lifestyle. This has been supported by experimentations. We believe that the theory will be accepted by more and more people in the near future.

Section Two: Reason for Getting Lifestyle Disease Is Change in Energy Path

I. Two Paths for Energy Metabolism

We have mentioned earlier about the three main reasons for lifestyle disease: eating too much, eating wrongly and lack of exercise. So what is the deeper pathogenesis? This comes down to the new theory of 'energy path' and 'energy conversion' which are put forward by us.

As shown in Figure Six, on the left side, two bending dotted lines in the centre represent blood vessel wall, the narrowest space in the middle represents blood capillary, the left side is artery, and the right side is vein. The food is absorbed into the blood by digestion and becomes blood sugar. The blood sugar moves through blood capillary walls and into interstitial fluid with the action of insulin, and further goes through cell membranes and into cells. This is the course of energy metabolism of blood sugar.

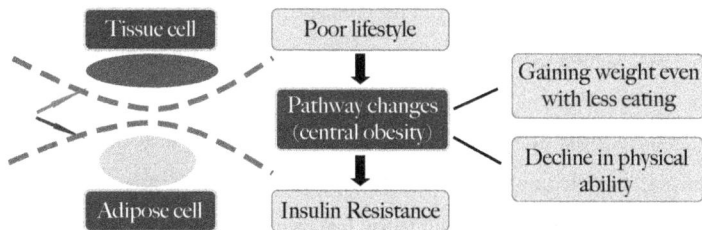

Figure Six: Conversion of Energy Metabolism

There are mainly two pathways for energy metabolism: one is transported to tissue cells, including skeletal muscle, internal organs, brain, immune system etc. to be turned into energy, physical strength and immunity. The other one is transported to adipose cells to store up. If it is reserved in the subcutaneous, it will develop obesity; if in the liver, fatty liver is caused; if in the blood, hyperlipidaemia and arteriosclerosis are resulted, and even causes myocardial infarction or cerebral infarction.

As for a person with normal metabolic function, the nutrition we intake are sent to tissue cells firstly, and sent to adipose cells to store up after it cannot be used up. Similar to a train which transports coal along the track, it meets a fork in the terminal. Normally, the railroad switch is pulled towards tissue cells. So, the energy can be continuously delivered to the tissue cells in the whole body first.

Whereas long-term poor lifestyle (eating too much, eating wrongly and lack of exercise) may increase the resistance of the normal path (towards tissue cells). Of which, including the increase of double resistance of capillary wall and cell membranes.

Firstly, look at the capillary wall. We have mentioned earlier that eating too much and eating wrongly will bring a lot of endogenous free radicals. They will firstly oxidize the weak capillary endothelium and cause inflammation. After the inflammation disappears, the capillary wall will thicken a little. It is similar to how the water pipe will thicken due to rust (caused by oxidation). The metabolic resistance which is met with when the insulin moves the blood glucose into thickened capillary wall will increase.

Then look at the cell membrane. There is a door in and out for glucose, which is insulin receptor. The receptor binding decreases due to lack of exercise. As if the door for glucose entering the cells is rusted, this will cause the increase of cell membrane resistance. Researches show that tissue cells may have metabolic disorders before adipose cells.

The track resistance brought by long-term poor lifestyle increases and accumulates continuously. The corresponding organs will secret more insulin to overcome resistance in order to move blood glucose to maintain its stability. Yet the accumulation of the resistance will reach a critical point at last, which will cause the railroad switch pulled from tissue cells to adipose cells, forming the change of pathway. This process takes about 10 to 20 years.

II. Fault of 'Insulin Resistance'

In the 1950s, Yallow and others applied radioimmunoassay to test for plasma insulin concentration. It had been found that patients with relatively lower plasma insulin had higher insulin sensitivity, and patients with relatively higher plasma insulin were insensitive to insulin, which put forward the concept of 'insulin resistance'. The finding of 'insulin resistance' demonstrates that there such metabolic pathway in human body does exist.

Insulin can promote the tissue cells to intake and utilize glucose. Or figuratively speaking, insulin is responsible for transporting blood sugar from blood into cells. 'Resistance' means that the increase of path resistance and decline in transporting efficiency of insulin give rise to inefficient use of blood sugar.

The critical of formation of insulin resistance is change of pathway. Namely the railroad switch is pulled from tissue cells to adipose cells. The most intuitive mark for pathway change is central obesity, shown through waistline expanding. For the yellow race, men's waistline is inadvisable to go over 90cm; women's is inadvisable to over go 80cm.

Once the waistline exceeds the dangerous red line, or once the pathway is changed, patients are bound to suffer from two troubles at the same time: gaining weight even with less eating, and decline in physical ability.

Why do we gain weight even if we eat less? We do not gain weight even if we eat more before 20 years old. Whereas nowadays, we get fatter even if we eat less. Why is this? Because the pathway is wrong! The energy is firstly transported to adipose cells to stock up. The more you eat, the more you stock up; the less you eat, the less you stock up. So no matter how much we eat, gaining weight is inevitable.

How about no eating? Someone lost 2.5 kg within a month with eating only cucumbers every day. But once s/he went back to normal diet, s/he regained 5kg. Why? Because the pathway has not been pulled back, once we start having meals (instead of being on a diet), it gives priority to reservation so the energy turns into fat. So, if we do not recover pathways, weight is certain to be regained after weight loss by any methods.

Why does the physical ability decrease? It is simple: physical ability can only be formed after the tissue cells get energy. Because the pathway is wrong, energy cannot be sent to tissue cells smoothly, which of course causes the decline in physical ability.

The condition is not resulted overnight, but formed over the past years, even several decades. So, if you find your waistline expanding, then you need to be careful. Because you may well be approaching to the critical point of pathway change and be starting to develop insulin resistance.

Hence, people should treat these small changes with great care, and check erroneous ideas at the outset.

Section Three: How Obesity Evolves into Triple H and CCVD (Cardiac-cerebral Vascular Disease)

I. Type II Diabetes Comes Uninvited

The insulin resistance may further develop into insulin resistance syndrome. The process is also how obesity (mainly central obesity) evolves into Triple H and cardiovascular and cerebrovascular diseases.

If we do not correct the fundamental problem of insulin resistance, the adipose cells in the stomach will also develop resistance to the excessive insulin, and tissue cells will release a lot of free fatty acids into blood. Then weight may not continue to increase, but the free fatty acids in the blood will destroy the cells of pancreas. Pancreas is the organ which produces insulin. The insulin level of patients start to drop, but the blood sugar level finally elevates. As a result, most of these patients will suffer from type II diabetes.

Since the appearance of insulin resistance, maybe it will take 10 to 15 years for you to suffer from type II diabetes (shown as Figure Seven). In the 10 to 15 years, it is found that the level of insulin resistance is rising (shown as the curve ①), and the blood sugar keeps stable (shown as the curve ②). The reason is that insulin secretion of patients is rising (shown as the curve ③) to adapt to the rising insulin resistance. As long as patients can keep secreting abundant insulin, the blood sugar will keep normal. Nonetheless, the process will cause the accumulated damage to islet cells. It will evolve into islet cell failure at last. The insulin secretions will suddenly go down after experiencing continuous rise, and the corresponding blood sugar will rise sharply, only at the moment you will be diagnosed with type II diabetes.

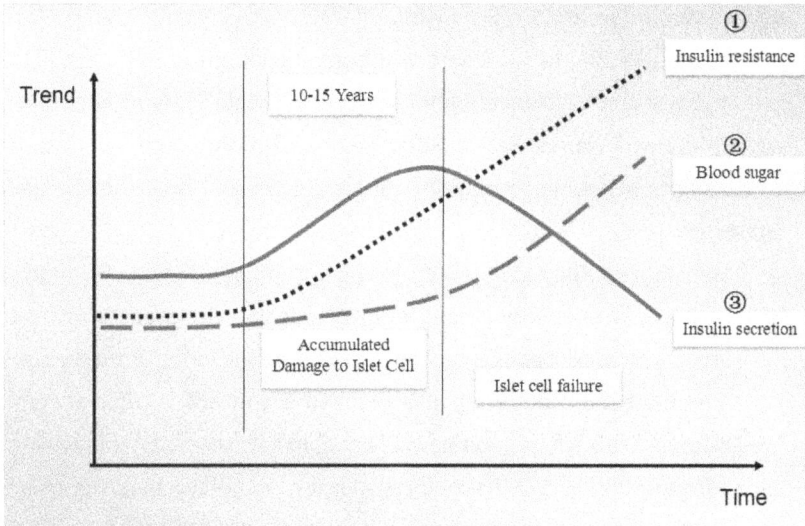

Figure Seven: The Accumulated Damage to Islet Cells

II. The Longer the Belt, the Shorter the Lifespan

Even if the weight does not increase any more, the fat will transfer from subcutaneous into internal organs, accumulate in the liver to form fatty liver, and enter into the blood to form hyperlipidaemia. The rise of blood fat will exacerbate blood viscosity, meanwhile the inner lining of artery is more likely to adhere to lipids to form atherosclerosis and finally cause clogged arteries. When it clogs the cerebral artery, it will cause cerebral infarction. If it clogs the cardiovascular, it will cause myocardial infarction.

The cerebral infarction or myocardial infarction are not formed overnight, but are accumulated over 10 to 20 years. The initial symptoms are cerebral anoxia and myocardial ischemia. So, if you are already obese, companied with dizziness, headache and amnesia, it suggests that you may well be in the early stage of stroke. If chest distress, palpitation and angina are always present, then you should start preventing myocardial infarction from now on.

It is a pity that most people will not take actions at this stage. That's why there are 80% patients with obesity and Triple H dying of stroke or myocardial infarction. Fortunately, more and more people have started to be aware of the seriousness of the problem, and seek the change of lifestyle.

Lifespan can be extended by losing weight and recovering pathway at this stage. Doctor Ray Strand pointed out that the process of insulin resistance can be reversed at any age, even after suffering from diabetes.

The medical community has reached a consensus: the longer the waistline, the shorter life you have. That is to say, the wider the waistline, the more visceral fat you have; the wider the waistline, the faster process of arteriosclerosis you have; the wider the waistline, the earlier you suffer from stroke and myocardial infarction.

The process of arteriosclerosis usually starts at a very young age for the modern society, and end our lives due to blocked blood vessel. So the medical community has reached a new conclusion: people have the same life with blood vessel. Therefore, it is more important to reduce waistline, but not lose weight for us.

Section Four: Discussion of Deeper Theory
(Selective reading for patients, compulsory reading for practitioners)

I. Free Radicals and Mitochondria

Oxygen is absolutely necessary for human. When human body makes use of oxygen, it will produce a charged oxygen molecule called free radical. The outer layer of the oxygen molecule has at least one charged unpaired electron. The high-activity oxygen molecule moves quickly and seeks an extra electron nearby. If the free radical has not been neutralized by antioxidant (it can provide an extra electron for free radical, which makes it harmless), it can continue to produce more free radicals.

In a complete cell, the mitochondrion is the centre of cell oxidative metabolism, and the place for the final oxidative decomposition of sugar, lipid and protein. Through the participant of O_2 (oxygen), sugar, lipid and protein are finally decomposed into H_2O (water) and CO_2 (carbon dioxide). In addition, protein also may form uric acid, urea etc. During the process, a lot of energy source ATP (Adenosine Triphosphate) will be produced for cells.

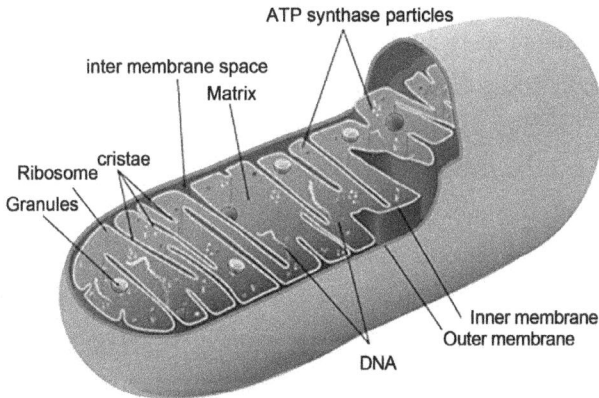

Figure Eight: Structure of Mitochondrion

The mitochondrion is a sensitive organelle which is the most vulnerable in the cells. Approximately 90% of oxygen inhaled by human body will be managed in the mitochondria. The mitochondrion (shown as Figure Eight) is a body of inner membrane wrapped by a smooth outer membrane. The breath of cells takes place in the folded inner membrane of mitochondria. When the breathing program is done quickly in the inner membrane, a lot of free radicals will be produced. This is the normal incidental in the process of oxidative decomposition.Over 95% of oxygen free radicals of human body are from respiratory chain of mitochondria. The first victims of free radicals are the inner membrane of mitochondria and mitochondrial DNA. This means that the mitochondrion itself is the most vulnerable part in the cell.

In the normal condition, these oxygen free radicals can be removed by antioxidant substance – SOD superoxide dismutase in the mitochondria. But with the aging of body, the activity of these enzymes declines, the oxygen free radical will accumulate in the mitochondria, which will cause the occurrence of various diseases. For example, the famous 'Keshan disease' is a mitochondrial cardiomyopathy, a disease of myocardial injury caused by the destroyed myocardial mitochondrial membrane due to selenium deficiency.

According to statistics, the accumulation from mitochondrion DNA oxidative damage caused by oxygen free radicals is 16 times higher than that from nuclear DNA. Mutation frequency of mitochondrion DNA is over 10 times higher than that of nuclear DNA. The nuclear DNA is the major genetic material in the cell, and has various kinds of restoration system to prevent DNA damage. Yet, mitochondria usually do not have such system. Therefore, the damage of oxygen free radical to mitochondria is more likely to accumulate and superimpose continuously. Many researches show that mitochondria are bound up with disease, aging, even probably individual life.

II. Blood Sugar Impact and Oxidative Stress

High-GI food will have an impact for blood sugar, and impact will bring more energy metabolism of mitochondria, then more free radicals will be produced in the corresponding respiratory chain. These excess free radicals will give rise to serious oxidative stress.

What is oxidative stress? Generally speaking, oxidative stress also can be called as the cell damage caused by free radicals. When the number of free radical increases, they will erode cell membrane, blood vessel wall, protein, fat, and even genetic material DNA. There are materials to resist free radicals in our body – antioxidants. Though, when there is no enough antioxidants, cell damage caused by free radicals will appear, this is 'oxidative stress'.

Scientific research has proved that oxidative stress is the fundamental reason which causes more than 70 chronic degenerative diseases, it is also the reason which induces coronary heart disease, cancer, stroke, arthritis and other diseases.

Let us recall, what causes high blood sugar impact? That is what we have mentioned above: eating too much (overeating) and eating wrongly (high-GI food, mainly refined rice and noodle) give rise to the fast rising of postprandial blood sugar, and make the increase in the number of free radicals noticeable.

For the sake of emphasizing: eating wrongly is the major cause of diseases.

Chapter Five: Self-Healing of Lifestyle Disease Using Human Instincts

Section One: Turn Internal Fat into Cellular Nutrition and Life Energy

I. Energy Conversion - 'Turning Waste into Wealth'

The pathological basis of lifestyle disease is the change of energy pathway. The key physiological method to cure lifestyle disease is energy conversion, namely how to convert fat in the body into cellular nutrition and life energy.

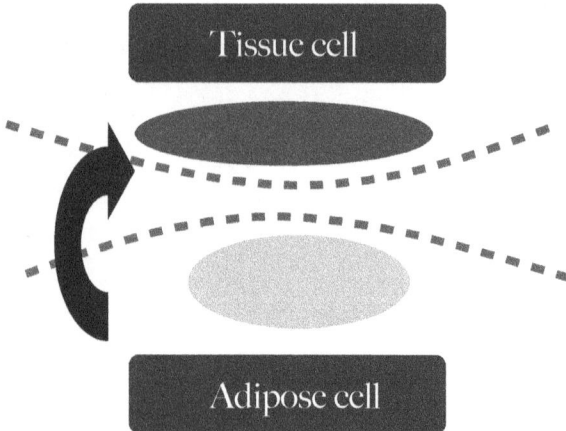

Figure Nine: Turning Waste into Wealth

One vivid phrase is 'turning waste into wealth' (shown as Figure Nine). We have drawn inspiration of human governance from the experience of environmental governance. The best strategy in the environmental governance is to turn waste into wealth. The so-called 'waste' is misplaced resource. As for petroleum, if it leaks into the sea, then it is pollution; if it is placed in the oil refinery, then it is resource. If too much fat is accumulated in the subcutaneous, liver and blood, then itis waste. But when it transported to tissue cells, it will be the nutrition and energy to restore cell function. Plenty of fat in our body are all nutrition we have once ingested, they are just misplaced. It is turning waste into wealth by delivering fat to cells.

In the process of energy conversion, a lot of trace elements are digested to ensure that there are enough coenzymes in the body to help the process of energy conversion, and the cells in the whole body will be activated quickly. Our organs are composed of cells, and every cell has the potential of self-healing. So, enough energy supply and a plenty of nutritional raw materials will facilitate the self-reduction of cells.

What is represented in the metabolism pathway is the regeneration and self-healing of tissues, namely self-healing of cell membrane and capillary wall. The resistance of the energy path to tissue cells will decline, and the switch will be pulled back again. So, energy conversion brings cell activation and accelerated recovery of path. Once the auto-metabolism recovers, human body will reduce or even get rid of drug dependence.

Energy conversion is a nutrition intervention on the surface, but actually there is an essential distinction between it and a general sense of nutrition intervention. Let's look at Figure Ten.

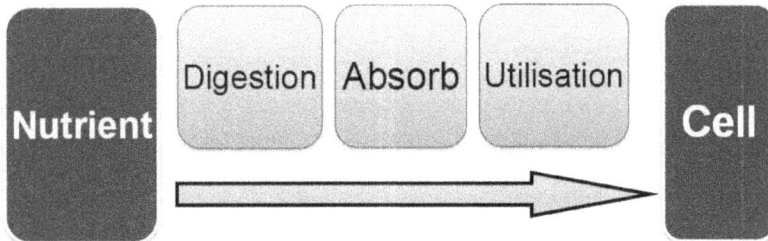

Figure Ten: Digestion, Absorption and Utilization of Food

The nutrition in the food will finally be delivered to cells. The process will go through three steps: first is digestion, mainly stomach participating; second is absorption, mainly intestines involved (take for spleen in Traditional Chinese Medicine); third is utilization, which requires the involvement of livers, it also involves all of the blood vessels, cell membranes, mitochondria etc.

Under special circumstances, cells need a lot of nutrition. For example, women can have 20 eggs every day during lactation period due to the need of cells. Chronic diseases also need a large amount of nutrition in the process of recovery. Cells in the whole body needs great overhauling and filling. So it needs a large amount of raw materials, which far surpasses the daily nutrition need.

However, in the conditions, cells usually cannot get enough nutrition. Firstly, you cannot have so much food, because the digestive ability of stomach is limited. Eating too much can only lead to indigestion. Secondly, the absorption ability is also limited. The excess food consumed is not possible to be absorbed fully, but possible to damage spleen and stomach for eating too much. So the limited ingestion and limited absorption finally result in that the nutrition moved to cells must be limited.

It needs to maximize raw material available to maximize the function of the self-healing ability of cells. While the general nutrition intervention can only provide limited nutrients to cells. So, it certainly limits the reducing speed of cells, and also limits the recovery speed of body. On the other hand, energy conversion can break through the limits of digestion and absorption of human body, and exert furthest the healing potential of human body.

Energy conversion directly makes use of third step: utilization. What we talk about turning waste into wealth is to skip digestion and absorption stage, and directly move the fats stored in the body to cells.

Fats are digested and absorbed nutrients that we have ingested.

Now we make direct use of it, and there is no limits of digestion and absorption. The general nutrient intervention is to obtain what cells can get, but energy conversion is to take such as cells need. To be successful in energy conversion, a combination of dietary nutrient and exercise is needed. Of which, nutrient intervention is a necessary part, but the key is a whole set of combined factors.

II. Magical Effect of Energy Conversion

The health improvement brought by energy conversion is all-around. In addition to the recovery of metabolism, it also includes the improvement of other two aspects:

On the one hand, the waste in the body is cleared up (namely the process of 'turning waste'), including the decline in subcutaneous fats, like the decrease of fats in the waist and abdomen, shoulder and back, hip, thigh, face and neck. What's more, it also includes the relief and disappearance of the symptoms of fatty liver (severe fatty liver also can recover), and the decline in the blood fat.

On the other hand, waste is turned into energy (namely the process of 'into wealth').

When the energy is moved to the bones, it will increase bone mineral density, and even improve the health of knees and hip joints.

When the energy is moved to the immune system, it will improve immunity, and accelerate improvement in various inflammations, like gastritis, enteritis and nephritis.

When the energy is moved to liver cells, it may improve liver function, raise the ability to detoxify, make your mood more comfortable and eyes brighter.

When moved to brain cells, it may improve thinking ability and memory.

When moved to skin cells, it may reduce wrinkle, tighten skin, and even change the overall shape.

When moved to the hair, it may make hair much thicker, have purer colour, and brighter.

When the energy is transformed into blood, it may make you have fuller blood, energetic and look healthy.

Even it may improve sexual function and boost the fertility due to the recovery of hepatic-renal function. For example, the female return to normal menstruation, or the menopause female restore menstruation; increasing the mobility of male sperm; after suffering from years of infertility, couples can have a successful conception by adjusting.

Section Two: Know Human Instinct Better Through Cells

Energy conversion is based on human instincts. The development of cell theory contributes to our further knowledge and understanding of human instinct.

I. Cells: Marvellous 'Little Things'

The human body is made up of cells. According to biological statistics, there are about 100 trillion (10^{14}) cells in an adult. These cells are divided into more than 200 different types. They also can be divided into over 600 types according to the extent of their cellular differentiation. There are big differences in their morphological structures and functions, but they all come from the division and differentiation of the first zygote.

The life of human is a multi-layered, nonlinear and multi-facet complex structural system. While cells are the basic units of the structure of living organisms and their activities. Completed life activities require the presence of cells.

The fundamental difference between the biochemical process in the cell and the process in vitro is that cells have a metabolism system with strict order and automatic control. The cloning technology further proves that every cell carry all information (called it as 'holographic function') of the life. The smarter human body has a magic and strong self-healing ability which cannot be replaced (even never be replaced) by technology, and the base for self-healing ability is the holographic function of cells.

As early as 1925, the biology master, Wilson, had put forward that all key questions of life could be found in the cells. The researches on major life phenomena like reproductive development, heredity and neural (brain) activities of living things should be based on cells. Similarly, physical rehabilitation and disease recovery also should be based on cells.

II. Structures and Functions of Cell

It is shown in Figure Eleven. A cell is mainly made up of cell membrane, cytoplasm, nucleus and organelles.

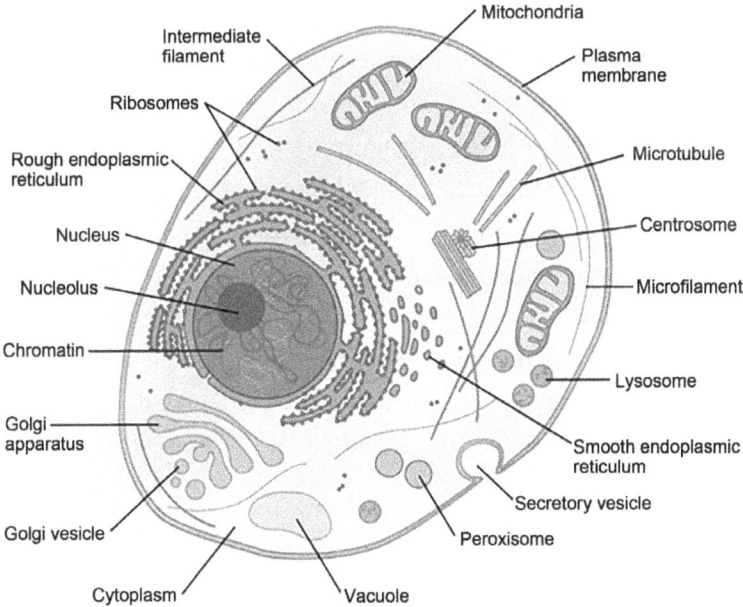

Figure Eleven: Cell Structure

1. Cell membrane

The cell membrane is biological membrane around the outermost layer of a cell, which is made up of lipid and protein.

The cell membrane is the boundary of the cellular structure. For example, cell membrane is like a territorial boundary of a country. Only when the boundary is stable, can the country have a relatively stable internal environment within the country.

There are many pathways in the cell membrane. They are just like the customs of the country. They are able to choose the useful nutrients to enter the cells and transport metabolic substances from the cells at the same time. These pathways also play a major role in energy conversion and information transfer.

The cell membrane is a membrane with fluidity, which is necessary for cells to finish several physiological functions. The fluidity of cell membrane depends on the lipids in the cell membrane. The more unsaturated fatty acid in the lipids, the greater the liquidity of membrane lipid has, and the more active the cell function is.

2. Cytoplasm

The cytoplasm is the substance located between cell membrane and nucleus. It contains nutrients which are necessary for cell growth, reproduction and self-healing. It is an important place for cell metabolism and material synthesis to take place.

3. Nucleus

The nucleus is the biggest and major cell organelle in the eukaryote. It is a storage place for genetic information and a regulation and control centre for cell heredity and metabolism. It is like the central core institution of a county.

4. Organelle

The organelle includes mitochondria, Golgi apparatus, centrosomes, ribosomes, lysosomes, and endoplasmic reticulum etc.

① Mitochondrion: it is the 'power house' of cells. It provides energy for various activities of cells. It is a place for final oxidation of sugar, lipid and protein.

② Golgi apparatus: it is the plant for sugar synthesis in the cell. Meanwhile, it processes, classifies and packages the protein, which are synthesized by endoplasmic reticulum, and then transports the protein to specific parts of cells or secret it to the outside of cell. It also can be said as a major transport hub for transportation of macromolecules in the cells.

③ Centrosome: it is the centre of internal activity while the cells divide. The centrosome ensures the symmetry of cell division process in mitosis, which is necessary for accurate separation of chromosomes.

④ Ribosome: it is the place for protein biosynthesis. They float within the cytoplasm or are attached to the endoplasmic reticulum.

⑤ Lysosome: it serves as the digestive 'organ' in the cells. Not only does it provide nutrients for cells; it also eliminates useless biomacromolecules.

⑥ Endoplasmic reticulum: it is the base for protein and lipid synthesis in cells.

We now have a basic understanding of the structure and functions of cells. Even though the knowledge provided above is shallow, we are still amazed by the wisdom of the Creator. The cell is an independent and real system which is 'governed by non-interference'. There is the nucleus that is in charge of general control, 'frontiers' -- cell membrane in charge of flowing and transferring the information and have selective input and output; the dutiful production department -- ribosome and endoplasmic reticulum; the 'power house' in charge of output of 'cell energy' – mitochondrion; also, it has its own transporting system -- Golgi apparatus; and the waste treatment system in the cells – lysosome. A small cell is just like a well-equipped factory. There are actually 100 trillion such 'factories' which are capable of highly self-management in a human body. They divide the work further, coordinate and function life in an orderly fashion.

Ever since the British Academic, Robert Hooke, observed slices of wood and described the cell structure of plants for the first time in 1665, scientists have always continually researched the structure and function of cells for hundreds of years. Since 1958, there have been total more than 60 scientists in the whole world who have the Nobel Prize because of their discoveries of cells and other related fields.

With the development of research, scientists have found that there exists a huge blank in the field of cells. Yet, something is undeniably true: even if it is a simplest cell, it is more exquisite than any current existing computer-controlled intelligence machine.

III. Stem Cell: Source of Human Body's Self-Healing

Each tissue of human body is able to renew by itself under the condition of the existence of adequate nutrients. It will take 5 days to grow a new intestine epithelium; 28 days to replace all skin cells with new one; 4 months to replace all of the red blood cells in the whole body; 6 months to replace all of the pulmonary epithelial cells; and 10% of bones are replaced every year. The ability to self-heal cannot exist without the powerful stem cells.

The stem cell is a cell with the potential of self-renewal, high level of reproduction and multi-directional differentiation. It is referred to as the 'all-purpose cell' in the medical field.

The human stem cells can be divided into two types: one is totipotent stem cells, which can be used for cloning human body directly; the other one is pluripotent stem cells, which is able to directly copy all kinds of visceral organs and tissues. Stem cells are just like dice. They exist in every tissue and organ in our human body. No matter what kind of cell our tissues or organs need, the stem cells will divide into such cell so they can play any role. Any disease is possible to be cured. The stem cell is the fundaments of humans' self-healing ability.

In short, even though technological exploration has made significant discoveries in many fields related to cells, the scientific understanding for two of the most basic and the most important questions still remains vague and ambiguous. One of the questions is how the lifeless macromolecule assemble itself into living cells step by step; the other one is how zygotes differentiate and develop into a complex human body.

Although we are unable to have an answer for these two important questions, one point is very clear: these are all human instinct. The science and technology are strong, but they are nothing when compared to instinct. We base the core idea of our rehabilitation scheme on stimulating the self-healing instinct.

Chapter Six: Nutrition and Exercise Are Main Means of Rehabilitation

Section One: Balanced Diet Is Necessary (I)

A certain condition is required for the human instinct to take place. As for the recovery of lifestyle disease by instinct, the most important condition is the balanced diet.

I. Basic Concept of Nutrition

The Father of Western Medicine, Hippocrates, pointed out that we should make food to be our medicine, but do not let medicine to be our food. The 'King of Medicine' in China, Simiao Sun, further pointed out that as a doctor, he should first know the source of the disease clearly, and understand how the patient has gotten ill, then treat it by diet. If it fails, only then the doctor should prescript medicine for the patient. The basic therapy on trend currently in the West also has the same ideology: for metabolism-related diseases, improvement in nutrition should be considered prior to taking medicine.

Why do human need to have meals? The general answer is hunger, but that does not mean that we do not eat if we are not hungry. Cells need nutrition, and thus human need to have meals. Specifically speaking, the nutrients are: protein, fat, carbohydrates, vitamins, minerals, cellulose and water.

Seven nutrients are the basic material of life. With the seven basic materials, thousands of biochemical components in the human body can synthesize by themselves. For example, myocardium which can obtain coenzyme Q_{10}, which is necessary for energy; endogenous antioxidant glutathione; protease for digesting meats; insulin for adjusting blood sugar, and estrogen for maintaining youth etc. As long as there are seven nutrients, these components can synthesize by themselves as required. (shown as Figure Twelve). When certain nutrients are lacking, the raw material which humans use for synthesizing are lacked, which will lead to various kinds of dysfunctions.

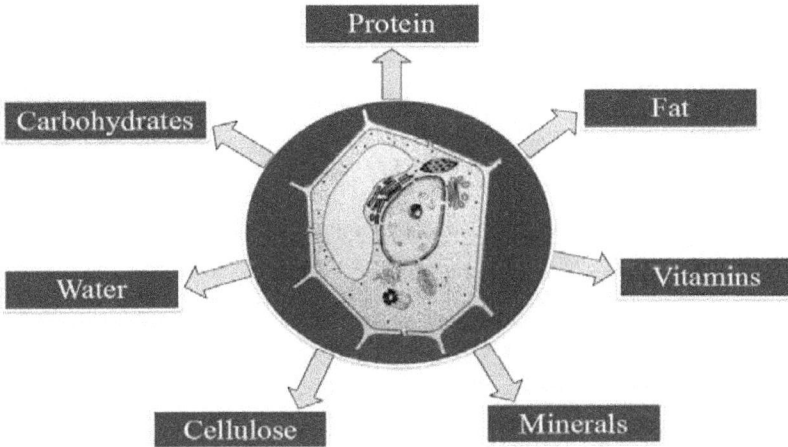

Figure Twelve: Essential Nutrients of Human Body

Looking at genetics point of view, nutrition cannot change genes, but can affect or even decide gene expressions. The same high-quality pine seeds, if one is planted in a fertile black soil, then it can grow into a giant tree; the one is planted in the poor soil, then it only can grow head-high. If the nutrients are lacking, the genetic function is unable to be expressed fully. Women are born with the genes to reproduce, but many of them are infertile due to malnutrition. Now imagine Michael Jordan, who has a great athletic talent in his genes, got rickets due to long-term calcium deficiency, development retardation due to zinc deficiency, anaemia due to iron deficiency, gastric ulcer due to vitamin B deficiency, and physical scars due to vitamin E deficiency after his birth. Even though he has a great athletic talent, it would not possible for him to become a great sport star.

The basic principle of nutrition is balance. Shown as Figure Thirteen, the balance is mainly the balance between three great energy sources (protein, fat and carbohydrates) and trace elements (vitamins and minerals). We can compare the three great energy sources to coal, trace elements are the oxygen which help the coal to burn. The more coal, the more oxygen the combustion needs. Trace elements are the coenzyme raw materials of energy metabolism. When having more meat, more vegetables are necessary to balance nutrition, or it is likely to get excessive internal heat (this is a concept in Traditional Chinese Medicine. Normally, people with excessive internal heat would easily get inflammatory, sore throat, toothache, acnes, etc.). The symptoms of excessive internal heat are usually the same symptoms as lack of trace elements.

When there are a lot of sport activities, not only more protein, fat and carbohydrates should be consumed for more energy, but also more vitamins and minerals should be consumed. Otherwise, the problems of vitamin and mineral deficiency, like muscle soreness, bone mineral density decline etc. will occur.

When the pressure and stress are great, the body will consume more calories. If trace elements are not supplemented immediately, the symptoms of trace elements deficiency, like baldness, bitter taste, mouth ulcer and light sleep etc. will be developed after the body is exhausted.

Basic Principle of Nutrition—Balance

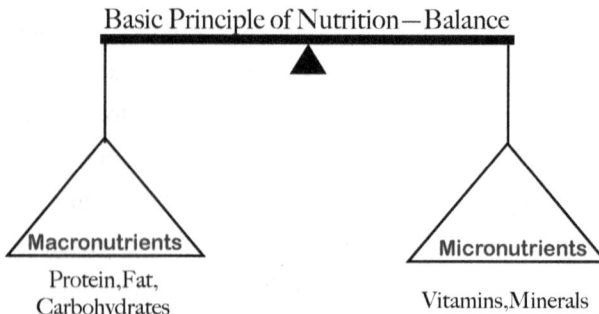

Macronutrients
Protein,Fat,
Carbohydrates

Micronutrients
Vitamins,Minerals

Figure Thirteen: Basic Principle of Nutrition

II. Understand the Seven Key Nutrients

1. Protein

Protein is the main composition of muscular tissues and all of the important internal organs. Protein deficiency will cause the decrease of organ functions, or even organ prolapse (such as gastroptosis, enteroptosis, anus prolapse, uterine prolapsed and skin laxity etc.)

Protein is also the main ingredient of enzyme, and enzyme is the catalyst for human body. If we were to compare a human to a light bulb, the enzyme is like electricity. Whether the body is full of energy or not is depended on whether the enzyme system is developed enough. Protein deficiency will lead to enzyme deficiency, which will cause decline in energy.

Protein is also the main ingredient for substances for immunity. Protein deficiency will lead to low immunity.

Protein is one of three great energy sources fir the body. In the extreme cases, like acute hunger, human body will dissolve protein by itself, and convert it into energy, like cutting the pillars of a house to light a fire for warmth in the cold winter.

The primary food sources of protein include fish, meat, beans, eggs and milk.

2. Fat

Fat is the main raw material for cell membrane, also the important carrier of cholesterol metabolism. As the energy is reserved, fat will be used as energy in the condition of carbohydrate deficiency. Fat is divided into saturated fat and unsaturated fat. The former comes from animal oils, whereas the latter comes from the seeds of plants, and fish.

In addition, it is worth mentioning that trans-fat is also unsaturated fat. Trans-fat is not necessary nutrients for body. It usually exists in the margarine, shortening agent and hydrogenated vegetable oil. Eating excessively will increase the chance of coronary heart disease. Yet, plenty of trans-fat is consumed despite the fact that it is not necessary for the body to consume.

Fat is made up of fatty acid and glycerine. From the perspective of physiological needs of body, fatty acid can be divided into non-essential fatty acid and essential fatty acid. The non-essential fatty acid can be synthesized by the body itself. The essential fatty acid is essential for body and cannot be synthesized by the body itself, so it needs to be consumed through food consumption.

Two families of 'essential fatty acid' are omega-6 and omega-3.

Omega-6: most people can obtain enough omega-6 from the normal diet. Its members include linoleic acid, y-linoleic acid and arachidonic acid. Of which, y-linoleic acid and arachidonic acid can be transformed by linoleic acid in the body. That is to say, the core representative of omega-6 is linoleic acid. It is the original member (mother) of omega-6 family. So as long as the linoleic acid is supplemented, others can be synthesized by themselves.

Omega-3: most people have deficiency of intake of Omega-3. It generally lacked in Chinese diet. The members include α-linolenic acid, EPA (Eicosapentaenoic Acid), DHA (Docosahexaenoic Acid). Of which, EPA and DHA can be transformed from α-linolenic acid in the body. That is to say, the core representative of omega-3 is α-linolenic acid. It is the original member (mother) of omega-3 family. So as long as enough α-linolenic acid is supplemented, EPA and DHA will be synthesized by themselves in the body.

The α-linolenic acid can prevent cardiovascular and cerebrovascular diseases, it changes the fluidity of blood platelet and regulates blood lipids. It plays an important role in adjusting insulin for diabetes. Meanwhile, it can protect eyesight and improve intelligence. Food which is rich in α-linolenic acid is shown in Figure Fourteen.

Percentage(%)

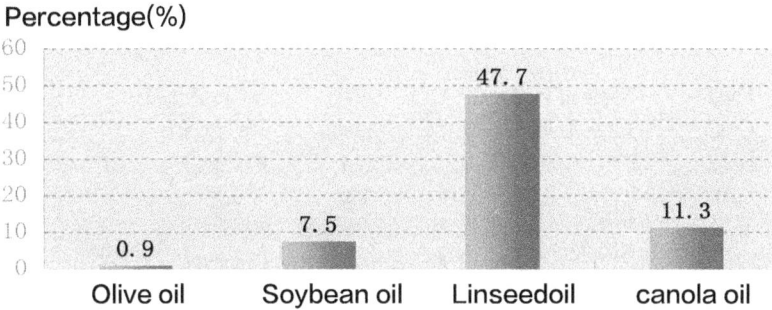

Figure Fourteen: Food Rich in α-Linolenic Acid

In summary, fatty acid is divided into non-essential fatty acid (there is no need to consume intentionally, it can be synthesized by itself) and essential fatty acid (need to be consumed through diet as it cannot be synthesized by itself). Additionally, the essential fatty acid is divided into omega-6 which are consumed in abundant amount, and omega-3 which is lacked and deficient, the key for the latter is α-linolenic acid

3. Carbohydrates (sugar):

Carbohydrate is the most important source of energy for human bodies. The primary food sources of protein include rice, noodle, fruit, sugar, tuberous vegetables etc. It can be simple carbohydrates (monosaccharide and disaccharide) and complex carbohydrates (starchy foods such as rice and noodle). The classification is done through the difference in their molecular structures.

If it is measured using GI (glycaemic index), legumes, dairy, vegetables (except for pumpkin, sweat potato, potato) and fruits (except for watermelon and pineapple) that we usually eat are all low-GI food. While there is a big difference for GI for different types of cereal. Usually, more highly processed the grain is, the higher the GI value. The high-GI food we intake in our daily life is mainly the highly processed grain (namely refined grains). Here are the GI values of some common food.

GI values of some common food

Food	Name of food	GI	Food	Name of food	GI
Grain and their products	Steamed buns (superior wheat flour)	88	Fruits and their products	Watermelon	72
	Rice	84		Pineapple	66
	Noodle	81.6		Mango	55
	Barley flour	66		Banana	52
	Millet congee	61.5		Grape	43
	Buckwheat noodle	59.3		Orange	43
	Brown rice	56		Apple	36
	Black rice	55		Pear	36
	Corn	55		Peach	28
	Wheat (cook the whole grain)	41		Plum	24
	Barley(cook the whole grain)	25		Cherry	22
Vegetables	Sweet potato (red, cook)	76.7	Legumes and milk products	Yogurt (with sugar)	48
	Pumpkin	75		Black soya beans	
	Potato	66.4		Lentils	42
	Chinese yam	51		Milk	38
	Cauliflower	<15		Tofu (stewed)	32
	Celery	<15		Mung bean	31.9
	Cucumber	<15		Soybean	27.2
	Eggplant	<15		(soaked then cooked)	18
	Celtuce (Chinese Lettuce)	<15			
	Tomato				
	Spinach	<15			
		<15			

4. Vitamins and minerals

Vitamins and minerals are both called as trace elements. They have the role of providing calories, but they are the raw materials of coenzyme in the process of calorie metabolism. Although the daily quantity demanded is only calculated by milligram or microgram, they play an important role of assistance and adjustment in all metabolisms. Meanwhil

-e, they also take part in constituting the human body, like bones, epithelium. Vegetables and fruits are the primary sources for vitamins; and seafood, dairy and bean products are the main sources for minerals.

Vitamin A: also called mucosal or epithelial vitamin. It can promote the secretion of mucus and protect mucosal system from bacteria, like nasal mucosa, respiratory mucosa, and digestive system mucosa. Vitamin A deficiency can easily cause dry eyes, dry nose, dry respiratory tract, dry legs, keratosis follicularis, rough skin, epithelial cancer etc. The causes of deficiency are air pollution and electromagnetic radiation from computers, TVs etc.

Vitamin B: also called as the coenzyme for energy metabolism. It can assist the metabolism of the three great energy sources (protein, fat and carbohydrates). Vitamin B deficiency tends to cause dry mouth, bad breath, glossitis, coated tongue, tongue cracks, cheilosis, dental ulcer, more nose oil, alopecia seborrhoeica, redness in the eyes, lack of power, muscular soreness and depression etc. The causes of deficiency are refined grains (Vitamin B family mainly exists in the bran of grains), great pressure and stress, too much calorie intake etc.

Vitamin C: the raw material of collagen. It is the 'welding point' to connect collagen molecules. Vitamin C deficiency tends to result in bleeding gum, periodontitis, purpura, scurvy and cerebral haemorrhage etc. The causes of deficiency are decline in food quality and the vitamin C may have been lost during the food processing etc.

Vitamin K: also called 'blood coagulation factor'. It can promote blood clotting and assist the calcium deposit in bones. Vitamin K deficiency tends to appear nose bleed, extensive haemorrhage, anaemia, haemorrhage during the menstrual periods and osteoporosis etc. It mainly comes from green leafy vegetables and personal synthesis of intestinal flora. The causes of deficiency are the disorder of synthesis of intestinal flora caused by using antibiotics; decline in food quality etc.

Vitamin E: lipid antioxidant. It can protect adipose tissues in the body from oxidation. When the fat in the blood is oxidized, the blood viscosity will increase. It will speed up the process of arteriosclerosis, cerebral infarction and myocardial infarction; when the cell membrane phospholipids are oxidized, large amounts of toxins will enter into cells to accelerate the cell senescence; when the subcutaneous fat is oxidized, it will form lipofuscin deposition, also called senile plaques. The causes of deficiency are decline in intake of vitamin E due to the refined processing of cooking oil, and use up more due to environmental pollution etc.

Mineral calcium: calcium deficiency tends to lead to osteoporosis, hyperosteogeny, spur, week teeth, soft fingernails, muscle spasm, face twitching, muscular weakness, fear of scare, neurasthenia, irritability, light sleep, Alzheimer's disease etc. The causes of deficiency are excessive intake of carbonated beverage, and less consumption of seafood.

Mineral magnesium: prevents bone spurs and calculi (stones), which are caused by calcium deposition, and relaxes muscles and nerves. The cause of deficiency is great intake of diuretic (tea, coffee etc.).

Mineral iron: the main raw material of haemoglobin. It maintains the normal hematopoietic function. Iron deficiency may be vulnerable to fatigue, sensation of chill, dizziness and powerlessness etc. The cause of deficiency is soil degradation caused by excessive use of fertilizers.

Mineral zinc: also called 'spark of life', it promotes production of new cells. If it is deficient during the brain development, it will limit the rate of cell division which affects intelligence quotient (IQ) growth. If it is deficient during growth, it tends to cause developmental retardation of height and sexual organs. It also will cause slow wound healing, leukasmus in nails, dietary bias and men's enlarged prostate etc. The cause of deficiency is soil degradation.

Mineral copper: assists the absorption of iron. Copper deficiency may be the reason of anemia, dizziness, fatigue, easy to be tired, tinnitus and giddiness etc. The cause of deficiency is also soil degradation.

Mineral manganese: assists the absorption of calcium. Manganese deficiency may cause congenital malformation, abnormal formation of bone and cartilage, impaired glucose tolerance and affect glucose metabolism. The cause of deficiency is soil degradation.

Mineral selenium: also called 'king of anti-cancer'. It may inhibit the growth of cancer cells. There is a better effect to take it with vitamin E and vitamin B together. The selenium deficiency is liable to cause baldness, too much dandruff, less sperms, cataract, myocardial necrosis, and chronic hepatic necrosis etc. The cause of deficiency is soil degradation.

Mineral chromium: the single impact factor of diabetes. It has the role of strengthening insulin activity. Mineral chromium deficiency tends to cause diabetes, arteriosclerosis and hypertension etc.

Mineral vanadium: can prevent cholesterol accumulation, lower high blood sugar, prevent dental caries and assist to produce red blood cells.

5. Fibre

Fibre cannot be digested or absorbed by the human body, but it is still listed as one of significant nutrients. Fibre is classified into insoluble fibre and soluble fibre.

The insoluble fibre can keep faeces (body waste) wet and soft. It is also called 'scavenger of intestines'. Because it can lock moisture in the intestines and keep faeces wet and soft, it can prevent haemorrhoids and anal fissure.

The soluble fibre can form sticky gel-like substance in the food and reduce the speed that food is absorbed into the blood, and thus slow down the impact of postprandial blood sugar. The soluble fibre is also an important nutrient for intestinal probiotics. It helps the intestinal probiotics to synthesize vitamin B, K and lots of immune substances.

Serious fibre deficiency is the main reason for the increase of colorectal cancer for the modern society. The primary sources of fibre are the brans of grains and part of vegetables. The cause of deficiency is refined grains so brans are lacked.

6. Water

Water is the main component of body fluid in human body, accounting for about 57% of body weight. It has the roles of temperature regulation, substances delivery, promotion of chemical reactions in the body and lubrication. The sources of water include boiled water, purified water, mineral water, spring water and biowater. Boiled water is a safe source of daily drinking water for most people. If it comes straight from the tap, the water purification and activation device can be considered to be installed for further improvement on the safety and activity of water. The purified water has an extreme high safety, but it lacks nutrients, like mineral. So, it is not recommended to drink purified water for a long term. Mineral water is manufactured by adding minerals to the purified water. Its nutritive value is higher than purified water, while its mineral activity is inferior to natural spring water. The biowater exists in the organisms. It has high biological activity, high nutritive value and other advantages. It is superior to all waters mentioned above. The methods of biowater intake include eating more vegetables and fruits, also include drink fruit and vegetable juice.

Section Two: Balanced Nutrition Is Necessary (II)

I. Other Great Factors of Naturopathy

In addition to seven nutrients, people find that there are other various valuable natural ingredients. We choose some of them, which have an important significance in treating lifestyle disease, to illustrate.

1. Oligomeric proanthocyanidins

Called OPC for short. It is a special bioflavonoid and an internationally accepted natural antioxidant which has the power to eliminate free radicals in the human body. The oxidation resistance of

OPC is 50 times as much as vitamin E and 20 times as much as vitamin C. Its main roles are as follows:

① improve blood circulation: Protect capillary wall, reduce capillary resistance and improve penetrability, which makes cells obtain nutrients and eliminate wastes much easier.

Professor Henrichoussat of University of Bordeaux, France, got 47 people (aged from 37 to 85) to take 100mg OPC in an experiment. Then it is found that the capillary resistance after 27 hours (of the intake of OPC) reduced by 40%. The experiment shows that OPC can reverse insulin resistance of capillary walls. In addition, it also can improve transport of electrolyte, and remove oedema. It also plays an important role in the heart. The fat intake of French people is far more than Americans. However, the incidence of coronary heart disease of alcoholics is 30% to 40% less than the people who do not drink at all. Because the French drink more red wine, which is rich in OPC. It can protect vision and reduce capillary haemorrhage in the eye group.

② skin beauty: OPC has a whitening effect. It can fade melanin and prevent lipofuscin from forming. It can synthesis of collagen and relieve skin problems, like wrinkles and cutis laxity. It has polyhydroxy structure. It can seize the water in the air to keep skin moisturized.

2. Oligosaccharide

It is made up of 2 to 10 glucosidic bonds and divided into functional and general glucosidic bonds. What has significance to human body is functional glucosidic bond. Its characteristics include difficulty in digestion and absorption, low sweetness and calories, does not increase blood sugar, and improves the growth of probiotic in the intestines. Of which, the most important one is the improvement on the growth of probiotic in the intestines, especially promoting the propagation of bifidobacterium. Bifidobacterium is the most common and the most important probiotic in the human body. It has an important significance in health. Its main roles are as follows:

① **biological antagonism:** Fermentation of bifidobacterium will produce lactic acid and acetic acid, which lowers the intestinal PH and inhibits the mycelia growth. So, it prevents enteritis, gastritis, and stool from stench, pox, fatigue and liver dysfunction.

② **immune regulation:** Inject bifidobacterium into the intestines of mice, after 2 to 4 weeks, bifidobacterium IgA antibodies is separated from the lymph, liver and stomach. It shows that bifidobacterium can synthesize large amounts of immune substance (about 70% of all immune substances in the body), which are delivered to the whole body to fully improve immunity and slow aging.

③ **lower cholesterol:** transform cholesterol into sterol that is not easy to be absorbed. Clinical trials show that blood cholesterol can be reduced by 50% during the period of taking bifidobacterium. This means that it can prevent arteriosclerosis and cardiovascular and cerebrovascular diseases by maintaining the health of the intestines for a long time.

④ **anti-tumour:** reduce the forming of carcinogens (amines, phenols etc.) in the intestines, and inactivate some cancer-causing enzymes. It can prevent intestinal cancer, gastric cancer, oesophagus cancer, breast cancer and carcinoma of uterus etc.

A survey on the Flora of Long-Lived People in Bama, published in 1985, shows that in the bodies of the long-lived people, bifidobacterium play a dominant role and its content is far higher than an average adult body. The filed survey done by Beijing experts in 1993 confirms that the content of bifidobacterium in the body of the love-lived people in Bama County reaches up to 1×108 -- 1×1010. The content of bifidobacterium of long-lived people aged 100+ is about 100 times more than the ordinary elderlies.

Alteration of intestinal flora manifests as foul smelling in bowel and dark defecate colour of faeces. The best way to improve intestinal flora is to consume oligosaccharide. The oligosaccharide has the promoting role in the growth of bifidobacterium, so it is called 'bifidus factor' and 'prebiotics'.

Common oligosaccharide includes isomaltooligosacharide, fructo-oligosse, soybean oligosaccharides and xylooligisaccharide. Of which, the function of oligosaccharide to xylooligisaccharide is 10 to 20 times as much as others.

3. Phospholipids

They include phosphatidylcholine (PC), phosphatidylethanolamine (PE) and phosphoinositide (PI). Phospholipids are widely used for the treatment of arteriosclerosis, liver cirrhosis and senile dementia in Europe and the US. Its primary functions include:

① the basic component of cell membrane: Phospholipids lose 5 to 8g naturally every day. The phospholipids deficiency will cause the low liquidity of cell membrane, and result in the decline in cell metabolism, including poor movement of nutrients in and toxins out. On the one hand, sufficient phospholipids can contribute to the repair of damaged liver cell membrane, promotion of regeneration of liver cells, continuously improvement on chronic hepatic injures (no matter what the cause is); on the other hand, they also can renew tissues of cerebral cell membrane, activate brain cells, relieve the degeneration and deaths of brain cells, boost memory and prevent Alzheimer's disease.

② emulsifying fat: by emulsifying big blocks of fat into fine granules for easy movement and to prevent fatty deposition. So, it can effectively prevent and treat fatty liver, liver cirrhosis and liver cancer; prevent gallstones (cholesterol crystal); remove the cholesterol deposition in the lining of arteries; improve brain oxygen; and prevent myocardial infarction, cerebral infarction and peripheral circulation disorder etc.

The human body can synthesize phospholipids by itself. Yet when the synthesizing function is damaged or the necessary nutrient from raw materials for synthesizing phospholipids are deficient, extra supplements are needed. The common food sources of phospholipids are soybean and egg yolk.

4. Carotenoids

It exists in the nature in the form of pigments. It is the main element that brings different orange or red for fruits and vegetables. Human has discovered more than 600 types of carotenoids so far. Of which, lycopene, beta carotene, alpha carotene, astaxanthin, lutein and zeaxanthin are considered to be relatively important. These carotenoids can transform into vitamin A in the human body and animal body. So it is also called 'provitamin A'. The excellent antioxidant property of carotenoids can protect plants from ultraviolet rays. For humans, carotenoids also can achieve excellent antioxidant effect. It also has particular value on preventing damage of free radicals, cardiovascular diseases and cancer.

5. Flavonoids

Flavonoid is also called bioflavonoid. It is the most abundant polyphenolic substance in the human diet. It widely exists in the fruits, vegetables, grains, rhizomes, barks, flowers, tea and red wine. So far, there have been more than 4000 different flavonoids discovered. Flavonoids can further be divided into:

Flavonol: such as quercetin, red onions have the highest content compared to other vegetables.

Flavones: such as luteolin and apigenin, it is contained in pimento and celery

Flavanones: mainly found in citrus fruits, such as hesperidin and naringin;

Flavonols: it is mainly catechinic acid, richest in green tea;

Anthocyanins: mainly the pigment in the plants, different level of content in different plants;

Proanthocyanidins: it is rich in grapes, peanut coat and pine bark;

Isoflavones: mainly distributed in soy food. It has been proved that it has a strong capability for anti-breast cancer and anti-osteoporosis.

The main functions of flavonoids include inhibiting the generation of harmful low-density lipoprotein, reducing thrombosis; holding back the degeneration and aging of cells, preventing cancer; improving blood circulation, lowering cholesterol, decreasing the morbidity of cerebrovascular disease and also improving the symptoms of cerebrovascular disease.

II. Meaning of Nutritional Supplement

Let's review the new version of the food pyramid. It is shown in Figure 15. There is a small bottle in the top left corner with text annotation 'various vitamins (most people)'. That is to say, for most modern people, it is the necessary for rational diet to supplement trace elements, like various vitamins, every day.

In addition to intaking nutrients from food combination, people also need extra supplements. Why are the supplements necessary? Isn't the proper diet enough to satisfy all nutrient needs of the body? What is the deep reason behind nutritional supplement?

Dr. Gunter Blobel, 1999 Nobel Prize Laureate for medicine, President of American Society for Nutrition, points out that the soil is poor now, and polluted by chemical substances like pesticides, herbicides, and acid rain, so all plants have lost part of native nutrients. When animals eat these plants, it is impossible to have enough the nutrients in their meat, milk and eggs. In this case, even though nutritionists understand how to combine food correctly, it is not possible to eat healthily.

The trace elements in the soil, which are necessary for various organisms, are now damaged. This affects the health of the whole biologic chain. As shown in Figure Fifteen, Ministry of Health and Welfare published the change of the content of vitamin C in 100g spinach from the same region with the development of history.

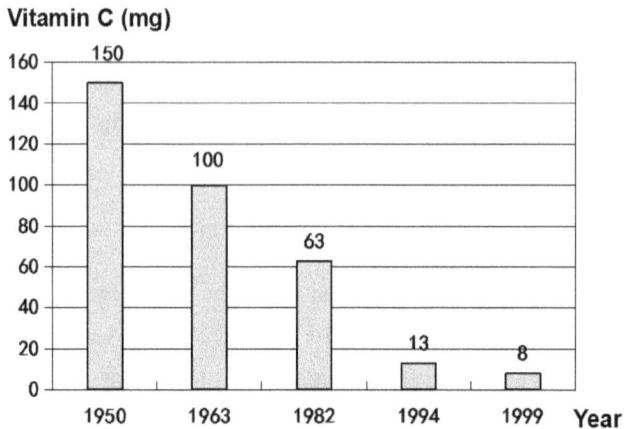

Figure Fifteen: Change of Vitamin C in 100g Spinach

German Black Forest Institute published a research report which compared the nutrients of the common food from 1985 to 1998, and recorded the changes in content. Of which, vitamin C in apples reduced by 80%; the content of magnesium in spinach had reduced by 69% from 1985 to 1998; the content of calcium in tomato had reduced by 71%; the content of folic acid and vitamin B6 in banana reduced by 87% and 93% respectively.

The poor soil results in the decline in the food quality, processed food result in nutrients loss, and environmental pollution results in the excessive consumption of antioxidant in the body. All three together have aggravated trace element deficiency of the global population. Consuming adequate nutrient supplement is a necessary component of healthy lifestyle, and important diet guiding principle of new Harvard food pyramid, it is also what protects us form diseases, ageing, sub-health, while improve our lives and standard of living.

The theory of energy conversion considers that nutrition supplement as an important role in the process of turning waste, or fats, into wealth.

On the one hand, once the body is in the state of energy conversion, extra fats stored in the body will continuously be converted into cell nutrients and life energy. It will cost more enzymes in the course than usual. So it's necessary to supplement multiple trace elements to help the human body to establish new nutrition balance. On the other hand, with the increase of metabolism brought by fat conversion, it is necessary to improve metabolic capability for each organ and tissue of the human body which are participating in the metabolism, in order to adapt to the new metabolic load. Examples of the functions which need to be improved: the defecation function of intestinal, the detoxification functions of liver and kidney, the function to move out more metabolic waste of cells etc. All these need an increase in nutrients, otherwise nutrition imbalance and metabolism disturbance will occur, which will result in problems in energy conversion. So other than daily nutrition supplement, it also needs further nutrition enrichment in the process of energy conversion.

III. Contribution of Modern Biochemical Technology

The development of modern biochemical technology makes a great contribution to dietary nutritional engineering, such as directed breeding technique, isolation technique and embedding technique etc. All these have very practical significances.

1. Directed breeding technique

The directed breeding technique has solved the problem since humans can now get a large amount of mineral with natural food. Taking selenium as an example, it exists as inorganic selenium (e.g. sodium selenite) and organic selenium (such as: selenium-enriched rice, selenium-enriched yeast etc.). The inorganic selenium has low absorption and utilization efficiency and greater toxicity, also the safety margin between toxic dose and nutritional requirement is small. The organic selenium is the selenium (sodium selenite) added in the process of cultivating the plant. It transforms from inorganic selenium into bioselenium in the natural food by making use of the absorption and growth of plant. The organic selenium (to be precise, bioselenium) has not only high biological activity, but also very safe.

2. Isolation technique

The isolation technique has solved the problem of purification and concentration of effective constituent in the food. Some specific nutrients in some food have special significance to human health. High intake of them may bring obvious physical improvement. For example, the phospholipids in soybeans have a special role in brain and liver; the OPC in black bean and grapes has extraordinary anti-oxidation effects; vitamin C, rich in the acerola cherries, has the role of improving immunity; the flavones in the oranges can improve blood pressure; and the polysaccharide in helianthus tuberosus Linn has the adjustment effect on blood sugar.

On the premise of preserving biological activity of natural nutrients, the techniques of isolation of distillation, extraction, ion exchange and crystallization etc. are able to improve the concentration level of nutrients by several times, or even ten times of its original level. So, the techniques help humans to digest more natural essence.

3. Embedding technique

The embedding technique protects special activity of some effective constituents. For example, vitamin E has a poor stability and is easy to be damaged by exposures to oxygen, ultraviolet ray, alkali and ferric salt. So, its utilization is limited. Vitamin E is made into microcapsule by embedding technique, which not only can keep the intrinsic property of vitamin E, but also can improve its stability and anti-oxidating property. In addition, the embedding technique has succeeded in pulverizing vitamin E oil. It is beneficial for storage, transportation and application of vitamin E. For example, probiotics are the active cultures which are necessary for the health of intestines. Yet, it is likely to be killed by gastric acid, so it is not able to enter the intestines through stomach. By embedding, probiotics are able to avoid damage from gastric acid with the protection of macro-capsule. So probiotics can now supplement beneficial bacteria for intestine.

Section Three: Have You Exercised Today?

In addition to nutrients, to play the instinct of the human body, it is also required to have regular exercise. The exercise we advocate is to combine movement and quiescent. The movement means aerobic exercise, and quiescent means meditation.

I. Movement Aerobic Exercise

The aerobic exercise means the physical exercise done in the conditions of sufficient oxygen supply. The common projects include: brisk walking, jogging, skating, swimming, riding a bike, practicing tai chi, dancing, rope skipping, doing rhythmic gymnastics etc. Four benefits of aerobic exercise are: controlling high blood pressure; increasing total blood volume; improving heart-lung function and increasing bone density.

On the contrary, anaerobic exercise (strenuous exercise) is easy to cause many damages to body, such as lowering immunity of human body; increasing cardiac load, and resulting in a heart attack; damaging sporting organs; accelerate ageing of the body, or even shorten human life.

Looking at cells, anaerobic exercise will increase endogenous free radicals, damage mitochondria and lower the energy conversion efficiency of cells. On the contrary, aerobic exercise will increase the number of mitochondria; moreover, it will improve insulin receptor binding of cell membrane. So it is conducive to reverse insulin resistance and recover normal metabolism.

Proper exercise contributes to health, which include:

1. Walking

'Hundreds of exercises are not better than walking'. We recommend walking as the first choice of aerobic exercise. Compared to other exercise, walking has three unique advantages:

① walking is especially good for heart health: Feet are the second heart of people. Because feet are the farthest away from heart, and the effects of gravity, blood is difficult to flow back from the feet. While walking, the speed of blood flow of feet increases. It is equal to adding a 'pump' in the farthest end of body, and it is able to help heart to pump blood back.

② walking is especially good for sleeping: The Chinese medicine pays much attention to diagnosis and treatment based on an overall analysis of the illness and the patients' conditions. Of which there is the concept of treating upper body diseases from the lower body. It contributes to solving the problem of brain when treating from the feet. Walking has notably outstanding effects on brain fitness, tranquilization, speeding up sleeping and deepening sleeping depth.

③ easy and convenient, and easy to be done: Walking is the simplest aerobic exercise. It can be done easily and naturally, and is not limited by time and place. It is convenient to do and easy to continue to do. Better exercise has no use if it cannot be done. So, walking is most likely to become one of the aerobic exercises for healthy lifestyle nationally.

The requirement of lifestyle disease intervention is two groups of brisk walking, over 15 minutes each, continuously every day until the back is heating up in order to maximize effects of exercise.

2. Fitness programs

All kinds of aerobic health fitness programs are also good choices. If place and condition allowed, you can choose a health fitness program which you enjoy, and dance several times every day. We recommend 'Wuxing Healthy Exercise' to you. It has a very good effect on all-around exercise and general recuperation. It is suggested to dance two sets every day, and 15 minutes per set. You can download the videos from the internet, and it is convenient to do the programs at home or in the office. Over time, you can do it anytime and anywhere without videos. It is

really very convenient and effective.

II. Still: Do Meditation in the Morning and Evening to Improve Potential

The same as walking, meditation is also a regimen that deserves to be stuck to for the whole life. The benefits of meditation are too numerous to mention one by one: relieve anxiety, tension, pressure and fatigue; improve the quality of sleeping; be more patient, caring and more harmonious to get along with people; clearer head, better memory, better creativity, keener observation and more delicate analysis; reduce one-track and parallel thinking way, be able to think broadly and fully and outside-of-the-box; balance Yin and Yang inside the body, and make the chi of viscera harmonious; fuller chi and blood.

When looking at cells, there are three remarkable effects from meditation.

① extend the cell division cycle: the division limit of human cells is 50 times, and each division period is 2.4 years. So the natural human life span can be prolonged by extending the division cycle. The relaxation due to meditation will bring the corresponding decline in breath, heart rate, blood pressure and body temperature. Researches show that low temperature will slow down cell division. So meditation can prolong human life by extending the cell division cycle.

② lessen cell respiration: meditation may lessen respiration of human body. It means to lessen cell respiration. The endogenous free radicals produced by the respiratory chain in mitochondria are the major reason to acceleration of ageing. Therefore, lessening respiration means reducing free radicals and slowing down ageing. Meanwhile, the chronic damage on mitochondria resulted from free radicals is the main cause to decreased cell metabolism. So, lessening cell respiration also means preventing humans from metabolic diseases.

③ reduce cell interference: science has proved that negative emotions like tension, angry, fear, anxiety will cause an increase of toxins in the body. This is means a large increase in the usage of cells, which causes a huge interference for cells to function normally. Meditation may eliminate various kinds of distractions, and help cells to maximize self-healing potential 'single-mindedly'.

In order to solve lifestyle disease, we advocate meditation to be a popular lifestyle. It is simple and easy to do, and also very important. The methods provided by the book are not aimed at guiding to cultivate and make elixirs, or immortality, nor the popular spiritual practice. 'Seekers are as many as the hair on an ox, but the enlightened is like the hair of a phoenix and the horns of a giraffe'. What the tedious and profound bring must be too complicated to be popular.

Below are several points related to meditation:

1. Time of meditation

① what is the best time for meditation? For the general meditation enthusiasts, both mornings and evenings are suitable. If only once is allowed every day, then the time when you wake up in the morning is the best. It is also effective to do a short period of meditation for 15 or 20 minutes before bedtime every night. In general, do meditation after getting up as first preference, or meditation before bedtime if mornings are not suitable.

② how to determine the duration of meditation? At least 30 minutes, at most one and a half hours. At the beginning of practice, we should do it at a higher frequency with shorter duration each time. When you are a beginner, a quarter to half hour each time is the maximum, then gradually increase the duration to an hour. For the beginners, meditation is not the longer the better. If you are terribly upset, and really cannot calm down with the help of meditation, you may as well get up and move around, and do something else. If you force yourself to stick to it, a sense of dizziness will come to you.

③ How to practice meditation during spare time? It is best to arrange a fixed time for meditation every day. When there are many miscellaneous things to do, and meditation cannot be arranged at the specific fixed time, then you may make use of your spare time. The specific method is:

Short-time meditation: about five minutes, it can be ended directly;

Relatively long-time meditation: more than 15 minutes, it is much better to be ended after doing breathing regulation (please refer to the 'Breathing regulation' in the section);

In a nutshell, because meditation is just to relax body and mind, there's not many deviations usually. The relaxation can be done at anytime from anywhere. Even one minute or two minutes is helpful and does no harm to body.

④ When should we not do meditation? It is not allowed to do meditation within half an hour after a meal; not during the female menstrual period; or after anger, you can only meditate after you are calm again.

2. Meditation environment

① How to choose the place for meditation? It is recommended to choose a quiet and well-ventilated place that is free from disturbances. Do not have your back facing the windows so you do not catch a cold.

② Dressing for meditation: Better to wear loose and comfortable clothes, take off tight clothes before meditation. Cover your knees with a layer of cloth to keep them from the wind.

③ How to choose seats? It is best to have a fixed and special chair for meditation. The chair shall be covered with a soft cushion so that your hip is 6 to 10 cm higher than your knees. For beginners with stiffer legs, the distance can also be 12 to 15 cm. If no special seats are available, you can also sit on a bed, but soft beds are not suitable.

3. Meditation posture

① What are the requirements when crossing legs? Many postures can be adopted while sitting with leg crossing, but there are three main types: two legs crossed, single leg crossed and downwards crossed. It is the best to sit with both legs crossed, and if this fails, sit with single leg crossed. For beginners who can't sit with even single leg crossed, sitting with legs downwards crossed is also advisable.

Two legs crossed: Put your left leg on your right thigh and make your left sole align with your right thigh, then put your right shank on your left thigh. At this moment, your soles are upward, and your thighs are cross with each other, forming a triangular shape.

Single leg crossed: While sitting, put your left shank on your right thigh, with your right foot under your left thigh. It is much easier to sit with single leg crossed than with both legs crossed. However as your left knee is not close to the cushion, your body will tilt left when you sit for a long time. If you immediately correct your posture when you find yourself tilting left, it does not matter.

Legs downwards crossed: It is also called loosely crossed. If you can't sit with either both legs crossed or single leg crossed, you can cross your shanks downwards. This is called legs downwards crossed. In this case, it is more likely for you to become tilted because your knees are not touching the cushion. So, it is advisable to adjust your posture immediately as soon as you find yourself tilted.

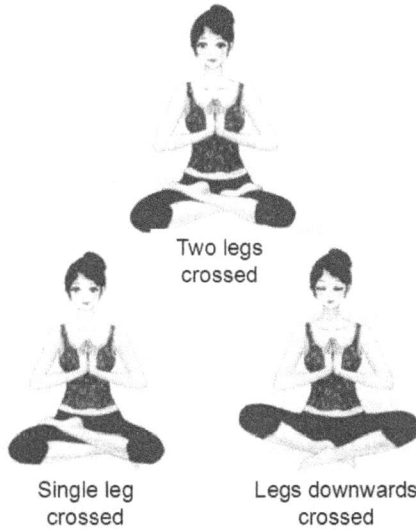

Two legs
crossed

Single leg   Legs downwards
crossed   crossed

② What to do when legs get numb? Beginners will feel that their feet get numb when they have been sitting for a while. When this happens, relax your legs and wait until your legs become not numb. Or stand up and walk slowly, then continue on with meditation.

However, it is better to not give up when you feel legs are numb and to tolerate it as much as you can bear. When you cannot bear it, you can interchange the positions of your both legs. If you cannot tolerate it anymore, give up and start another meditation after relaxing.

③ Head posture: Meditate with a smile, not laugh. Just to relax your facial muscles as well as facial neuroses. When your facial neuroses are relaxed, you become relaxed. It is better to close your eyes, as your mind will get tranquil with your eyes closed. Eyes closed, or more like have your eyelids dropped. Have your eyelids naturally dropped but not tightly closed. Lightly close your mouth, with your upper teeth slightly separated from lower teeth, and tongue against palate.

④ Body posture: Make your cervical vertebra straight and relaxed, but not stiff. It is important to have your chin slightly backwards.

Straighten your spine, but not lift your chest. Make your spine straight naturally, but no like a pen.

The weight of your body should be put between your thighs, but not on your hip. Therefore, your body is not at 90 degrees, but is slightly forward, with your weight in the centre.

⑤ Hand posture: Sit with your hands relaxed without any force applied. Put the back of your right hand back on your left palm and then gently put your hands on your shanks and close to your abdomen.

4. Breathing regulation

① Regulation prior to meditation: Adjust your sitting posture, have your hands before your abdomen, your upper teeth slightly away from lower teeth, your chin slightly backwards, and spine natural straight and upright. Breathe out waste air through your mouth from your abdomen and breathe in fresh air through your nostrils to your abdomen. Take subtle, smooth and even breaths for three times to the extent that you can achieve even breathing, and then breathe at a constant pace.

② Regulation during meditation: Breathing counting is a breathing regulation meditation that combines breathing and consciousness. Make your breaths subtle, slow and even, and then begin to count. When you are counting, whether breathing in or out, count from one to ten and then repeat, or from one to twenty, or even to one hundred. However, no matter how you count, you should restart counting if you miscount or are interrupted. In this way, as time passes, you will have regulated breaths and a peaceful mind. During meditation, you should correct your sitting posture when you find yourself not sitting straight.

③ Regulation after meditation: Take three deep breaths as what you do prior to meditation, breathe out through your mouth first and then breathe in through your nostrils. Then warm up your hands by rubbing them against each other, and wash you face with your dry hands from bottom to top. Next, rub your ears with your index fingers and middle fingers and then comb your hairs with your dry fingertips from the front to the back. Finally, open your eyes.

When you are disturbed during the meditation, do not open your eyes immediately. Take a deep breath first, and then open your eyes even though you can't complete the breathing regulation before finishing the meditation.

To sum up in a few words:

Meditation also follows our most important principal – simple and easy to do. What mentioned above were the most important points in the fewest words. To be even simpler, then there is only a very important point—sit.

If you do not sit, all other points are pointless. As long as you sit crossed-legged, maybe only for one minute and without doing anything as mentioned above, the chi and blood will be improved, and fatigue will be relived. Meanwhile the habit will be established gradually, and other procedures (as mentioned above) will be carried out step by step. Look for chances to have a sit at any time, from anywhere. A few minutes, more than ten minutes, tens of minutes, it does not matter, they are still better than nothing.

If the first step is done and you do meditation every day, then what is the next important step? That is sitting straight. While sitting, all tricks like keeping orifices, directing your chi, dead-cat bounce, and thinking about elixir field, are not necessary. As long as your body is upright and still, it is the best. It can be simply summed up as having your body loosened but straight. It is neither rigidity, nor floppiness. Because rigidity is against relaxation and floppiness goes against the self-moving of Chi.

If we can keep doing meditation every day, and keep upright while doing it, then what is the most important thing to remember during the process of meditation? Breath-counting. A strong thought can eliminate all weak, useless thoughts. Breath-counting may remove distractions. Meanwhile, breath-counting is the best breathing method, and the best way to gain calmness.

Chapter Seven: 'Cell Comprehensive Revitalisation Program' -- Simple and Effective Package Solution

Based on the principle of getting rid of the complicated while keeping the simple, and aiming at the masses, through long-term study, reflection, practice and correction, we have established a set of systematic solutions – Cell Comprehensive Revitalisation Program. The program chooses the simple and effective essentials in the lifestyle as means, has the purpose of taking care of human instinct, and meanwhile pays attention to the establishment of long-term habits.

Section One: Establish Basic Strategy

I. Pay Equal Attention to Thinking and Behaviour

The change of thinking will lead to the change in behaviour. The people, who have had thinking training, have more active and more self-conscious behaviour. They are more likely to resist distraction, to more likely to follow behaviour codes, and change their lifestyle for the better. In turn, the change of behaviour will lead to the change in thinking. People understand better due to success. They are more convinced due to experience. They have a greater understanding of theory due to practice. In order to naturally carry out thinking and behaviour training, we have adopted the methods of establishing training camp, setting up coaches and establishing reinforcement training camp.

1. Training camp

The training camp is the most effective comprehensive education platform. It includes thinking training: expert instruction, sharing with all class members, group discussion, and representative speech, reply and examination. Trainees are graded and awarded as a group. It also includes behaviour training: food plans, extra meals, exercises etc. It is aimed at starting the implementation of by program by comprehensive and systematic education.

2. Coaches

Through a lot of experiments, we have established a systematic, professional and generalized private coach pattern. The coach will continuously carry out thinking and behaviour training in the process of one-to-one private training.

3. Reinforcement training camp

The trainees who have had the camp once will have strong perceptual knowledge due to a great number of physical improvements. Yet the perceptual knowledge can only be enduring if it is developed to rational knowledge. So the further education in the reinforcement training camp is to help the trainees to change their lifelong thinking and behaviour in order to reach true health with no outside help, and finally have health and long lives.

II. Pay Equal Attention to the Individual and the Family

Human is the foundation of the medicine, so individuals are very important. Meanwhile, family is the most basic unit of the society, and the most important carrier of life and culture, so family is also very important. The family members are the closest to us, they care about us the most and have the most influences on us. When they cannot understand, they will interfere and disturb us out of love. It has been found that one family may have mutual effects and interactions on each other when living in the common living space. The effects of collective performance are always better than individual performance. So we advocate that family members may reach a consensus to take part in the management scheme of which is to re-establish lifestyle, and they may establish and pass on the family healthy culture as well.

III. Pay Equal Attention to Short-Term and Long-Term

The short-term schedule lays a foundation to the establishment of long-term habits. Whereas the establishment of long-term lifestyle consolidates the effects from short-term nursing. If we only pay attention to short-term schedule, and ignore then long-term schedule, then weight regain and Triple H relapse will occur. If we only focus on the long-term schedule, but ignore the short-term, people will give up because they do not see effects quickly

Section Two: Basic Principles of Plan-Making

In order to satisfy the need of the majority of the population, the schedule must satisfy three great principles: effectiveness, simplicity and comfort.

I. Effectiveness

Reasonableness is pointless when there is no effectiveness. The effects should be present for a long term. Patients care about that whether if the weight will be regained and Triple H will reoccur or not. The only long-term solution for this is to eliminate the main cause for concern, which is poor lifestyle. So the program shall be a long-term plan. It not only manages obesity and Triple H in the short term, but also establishes long-term habits.

Moreover, it has to have rapid effects. It is clear from experience that new lifestyle is always difficult to be re-established, and many attempts often fail. A driving force is necessary to turn short-time attempt into long-term behaviour. The driving force mainly comes from visible effects. So, the short-term program must intensify the effects to give the patients hope, build up confidence, so they would keep trying.

From the general attitudes of the modern people, the significant effects need appear within one to three days, including effect that can be monitored by clinic and can be perceived by themselves, so as to reduce the probability of patients giving up halfway through the treatment to the utmost extent.

II. Simplicity

The modern society has fast-paced life, and generally needs much simpler programs. If more areas are covered, the treatment is more complicated, then it is less doable or achievable. A program is nothing if it cannot be implemented, no matter how great it is. The patients, who are made a doctor because of the long-time illness, always say that 'I know all experts claim, but I cannot do it because it is too complicated and troublesome'. So, an important topic when coming up with the program is simplicity. We even sacrifice effects for the sake of simplicity. We have deleted the steps in the treatment which have little to no effects, and simplified the steps, which have a big influence on the effects, in order to make program easier to operate. The final result is that we have come up with a solution which can be understood as soon as it is heard, and it can be learnt quickly. Everyone can accept it and carry it out anytime and anywhere.

III. Comfort

Many people decide to lose weight, but they are defeated repeatedly because they cannot endure the temptation of the delicious food or cannot bear the pain brought by tiring and intense exercise. Many Triple H patients have once been serious about changing their own life. Yet they cannot eat most of the things during the change, and finally realize that 'there is no purpose of living if we were to live like this', so they will indulge themselves occasionally. The methods that go against humanity cannot be used for a long term. For the sake of maximizing utility, the program must not be difficult. Being healthy shall be a happy journey. Comfort means being both deliciousness and healthy, it should both improve obesity and Triple H, and have physical and mental pleasure.

Section Three: Core Contents of the Strategy

'Cell Comprehensive Revitalisation Program' includes four sub-programs: short-term program, long-term program, aided program and other habits. Of which, the most important are short-term program and long-term program. The aided program is a set of selective plans targeted at special people. The importance of other habits is inferior to the three great habits established in the short-term program and long-term program, but it also has a certain effect on lifestyle disease. If it is implemented appropriately, the improvement effect will be further enhanced. Overall speaking, it will achieve the most appealing effects by strictly carrying out the full set of the program; or only achieve part of effects if the program is carried out partially.

I. Short-term program

The short-term program is a set of enhancement plans. It aims to regulate metabolism, knock off extra pounds, restore to a healthy weight and recover the original metabolic functions of blood glucose, blood pressure and blood lipid. One cycle of short-term program is 42 days. Many cycles can be implemented one after another. The main contents of the short-term program include the following three points:

1. Low carbohydrate diet

It mainly restricts food which is heavy in sugar, like staple food. Other low carbohydrate diet can be digested normally, like various kinds of protein (fish, meat, soybean, egg, milk etc.) and vegetables (except for the tubers and vermicelli class). Sugar is the primary source of energy, fat is energy reserves. As long as the diet contains enough sugar, our body will give priority to choose sugar for the supply of energy for cells. When the intake of sugar is limited, body will start using energy reserves – fat to supply energy for cells.

2. Nutrition enrichment

The plan supplement multiple trace elements and comprehensively strengthen necessary nutrition for cells. On one hand, this provides enough coenzyme for fats to be transferred into cell energy; on the other hand, this provides abundant raw material for self-healing and reconstruction of the functions of the cells.

3. Action combination

Aerobic exercises, like brisk walking or aerobics, are done at least twice a day with over 15 minutes each. Also, at least one 30-minute meditation every day.

The key of the short-term program is not just one of the steps, but the combination of all three. If there was only low-carbohydrate diet but no nutrition enforcement, various kinds of nutrient imbalance would occur, like constipation, alopecia, bad breath, muscular soreness, lacking in strength, cramping etc. If there was only nutrition enforcement, but no low carbohydrate diet, it will not start changing the fats into 'wealth'. This means that not only is there no weight loss effect, but also the recovery of blood glucose, blood pressure and blood lipid is slow. If there was only low carbohydrate diet and nutrient enforcement, but no regular exercise, it goes against the activation of cells in whole body, and the effect of losing weight will be reduced. It will be not ideal for the rehabilitation of Triple H.

II. Long-term Plan

The long-term program is aimed at maintaining a suitable level of metabolism for a long time, and preventing weight regain and Triple H recurrence for life by establishing right lifestyle. The main points are as follows:

1. Low glycaemic index diet: eating less refined grains, and more coarse grains;

2. Supplement daily nutrition: supplement various kinds of trace elements, which may be deficient generally due to the declining food quality.

3. Action combination (exercise and meditation) and keep doing them.

It may achieve radical reform by combining short-term program and long-term program. The short-term program rectifies: restore body's own function and get rid of drug dependence; the long-term program takes a radical reform: establish right way to live and eliminate the causes.

III. Supplementary Plan

Aided plan is a set of plans of intestinal detoxification and blood clean. The main thing is to drink more than 2500ml of fruit and vegetable juice (apple and carrot at a ratio of 1:1) to replace the whole day diet, and appropriately cooperate with nutrient enrichment. The plan is suitable for two types of people:

People with excessive intestinal toxins: the plan clears up intestinal and blood toxins, create pure body liquid, and create conditions for cell to absorb nutrients.

People with relatively worse hepatic and renal function: the plan solved the problems of high uric acid, high urine protein, it reduces the liver and kidney load and accelerates the regeneration of liver and renal tissues.

The aided plan can be used by itself, but also can be used with short-term intensified program. The duration of the plan is flexible, as short as 1-3 days, as long as 1-3 months. The most commonly used are one-week small cycle and one-month great cycle.

IV. Other Habits

1. Sleeping

Once the short-term program is implemented, the sleeping quality will be improved quickly. So, what we need to emphasize is sleeping time. Firstly, ensure to sleep before 10:30 pm. Enough sleep will make you energetic and make your cells active. More active cells will consume fat more quickly. So, the better the sleep, the more energetic the cells are, the faster the fat burns and the more obvious the improvement of Triple H. In addition, it will cost protein to stay up late. Although it will bring to a thinner body, it also results in the decline in muscle and cutis laxity. So, staying up late will reduce the lean meat, while good sleep will reduce fats. Secondly, go to bed if you feel sleepy. Once the energy conversion starts, it starts the overhaul of whole body. Most people will feel sleepy like a baby. The body develops faster when sleeping, which means that the cells of the whole body grow and renew faster. Go to bed if you feel sleepy, which is just in order to better coordinate the heavy overhaul work of the whole body.

2. Drinking water

It is listed in the short-term program that every trainee needs to drink 2400ml of water every day. It can be mineral water, boiled water, purified water or activated water. In short, it must be sugarless. Whereas, for the long-term program, 2000ml of water is needed every day, it is also ok to drink fruit and vegetable juice, as well as sugarless drinks. The short-term program needs more water, because cells will produce more waste in the process of energy conversion, and needs more water to clean it up. Otherwise, waste accumulation will be slow down fat combustion.

3. Nuts

A handful of nuts every day increases the intake of good fats. Good fats are relatively deficient in our dietary structure. There are two basic ways to increase the intake of good fats: one is eating more fish and less pork, beef or lamb; the other means is to choose linseed oil or olive oil for cooking. It is also acceptable to use other pressing vegetable oil, but not refined oil.

No matter if you have done above two basic methods or not, we suggest that everyone should develop the habit of eating a handful of nuts every day. On one hand, nuts are rich in natural vitamin E, so they can protect the heart and are anti-aging; on the other hand, nuts contain plenty of good fats. It can reduce blood lipid and prevent arteriosclerosis. Hazelnuts, walnuts, almonds and cashews are referred to as 'The World's Four Great Nuts'. From both the nutrition and taste points of view, they are the best among all kinds of nuts.

Section Four: Application of Traditional Chinese and Western Methods in the Plan
(Selective reading for patients, compulsory reading for practitioners)

Traditional Chinese Medicine (TCM) and Western Medicine each has its own characteristics. They are both the wisdom essence of human's long-term struggle with diseases. They both make a great contribution to the establishment of modern medical system and extension of the average lifespan. Their differences are because of the differences between Chinese and Western cultures.

The core of Western Culture is self-cognition, whereas the core of oriental culture is unity of nature and man. It is reflected in politics: western society pursues for the people-oriented democracy, while the oriental community goes after the Great Unity of integral harmony. In the medicine, Western Medicine forms the concept of instinct, and emphasizes the talents and potential, and focuses on the understanding human body. On the other hand, Chinese medicine forms holism, establishes yin-yang and the five elements (metal, wood, water, fire, earth), midnight-midday ebb flow, health preserving in the four seasons and other systematic methods. The Western Medicine focuses on real evidence, more like a science; Chinese Medicine emphasizes dialectic, more like a philosophy.

Is the Cell Comprehensive Revitalisation Program Chinese Medicine or Western Medicine? It should be said as neither, but also both. We do not start deriving the plan with either the Western Medicine or Chinese Medicine, but we focus on solving the problem. As long as it beneficial for solving the lifestyle disease, when it needs TCM, then we use TCM; when it requires Western Medicine, then we use Western Medicine; when it needs education, then we use education. If necessary, we also can combine them together.

I. Application of Western Methods

The main Western methods are medicine and examinations.

During the early stage of the treatment, blood glucose-lowering medication and blood pressure-lowering medication are still compulsory, however, the amount can be reduced as the functions of the body recover.

Take blood glucose-lowering medication as an example. We first reduce the amount of the night dosage, then the morning dosage. We first reduce the amount of short-term medication, followed by the cut in long-term medication. The extent of the cut in dosage depends on the recovery of the body. If the function of the body of lower blood-glucose improves, but the dosage for medication is not cut, then low blood sugar may occur. Additionally, although some people may be off medication quickly, however, relapses may occur. If so, some medication can be used to assist with lowering the blood sugar.

There is a process for the recovery of human instinct. It is normal for some fluctuations to appear. The application of other drugs is similar to this. If drugs are not necessary, then no drugs are used. Only use the drugs, which specifically control the indexes needed, to control the specific indexes. The change of dosage should aim to stabilize the indexes.

The test for the conditions of the body is routine physical

examination. This includes the conventional indexes that reflect lifestyle disease, like blood lipid, blood pressure, blood glucose, uric acid, weight, fat percentage and waistline. Of which, blood pressure and blood glucose should be tested every day to be used as a guide for change of dosage. Other indexes can be tested before and after the short-term program.

There are two limitations of our test method: one is that it is not good at doing other comprehensive physical examination programs other than the lifestyle disease examination. Although, most of the time, the patients do a more comprehensive physical examination elsewhere without us intervening, and often find more health improvements on other aspects, so far it is unable to complete a systematic discussion on broader health problems. Second limitation is that there is lack of data of other indexes related to lifestyle (other than blood glucose and blood pressure) which describe the changes during the short-term program. So, we only know the change before and after the short-term intervention, but we have lack of quantitative descriptions of the change during intervention process. We ask for more participation from more medical institutes, they should exploit their medical advantages, and accelerate the resolution of lifestyle disease.

II. Application of Traditional Methods

The application of TCM (Traditional Chinese Medicine) mainly reflects in the food classification and therapy.

The food combination in the program is based on the classification and quantitative calculation of nutrition. This is effective on most people. For a few people with very special physique, the food combination is calculated by food classification and TCM. The people, who appear to be deficient in yin during the process of implementing program, tend to be given food which nourish yin (including meat, vegetables and fruits). Vice versa for yang. Sometimes, we also specifically choose some soup and diet, on condition that it meets the quantitative requirements of nutrition.

We have applied acupuncture, moxibustion, fire therapy, foot bath of Chinese Tradition Medicine and other traditional Chinese therapy in practice. The main purpose is not to accelerate the rehabilitation of metabolism problems, like obesity and Triple H (of course it is also helpful, but the program already has very obvious effects), but to strengthen the targeted treatment in other special problems. Experiments show that appropriate application of TCM therapy methods is especially good for alleviating the symptoms of side effects (in TCM, these are some discomforts caused by the treatment, but may not necessarily mean a worsened condition) and accelerating the disappearance of side effects. Although the work we have done on this is not systematic enough, we have confirmed that TCM therapy methods contribute to utilization of human instinct.

The medical research still has a long way to go. We hereby welcome front-line TCM workers to participate in our practice more, and make the great and profound TCM to contribute more in solving the lifestyle disease. Meanwhile, we suggest that we may combine systematic specialist treatment with lessons of simple regimen. Not only does it bring health for more patients, but also strengthens TCM.

Part Two: Practice Experiments

So far, a great number of experiments have given us two clear conclusions. First, Cell Comprehensive Revitalisation Program is effective when solving lifestyle disease; second, the stricter the implementation of the program, the more ideal the outcome.

It is undeniable that there have been some cases and experiments that are not as successful, and in some cases, have failed, but most of the cases have achieved great success.

After reflection, the reasons for the failure of the practice re as below:

1. Individuals: some patients are very old (i.e. 70 years old+), and have been sick for quite a long time (i.e. more than 20 years), which have had a few effects on the improvement results. There are some who are not that old and with short period of sickness, but they have used hormones for treatment or have removed organs (such as the uterus, ovaries), so the effects are not as great. There are also a few who did not have the problems as mentioned above, yet they lose weight very slowly (recovery from Triple H is, however, not slow), which suggest the presence metabolic disorder.

We don't have the solutions to the failure (or not so successful cases) caused individuals, so we can only persuade the patients to accept the truths.

2. Method: we have designed both quick and slow solutions. The slow one is more lenient, with no limits to the amount of vegetable and meat they take. The quick solution is strict in the food intake but different varieties of food are allowed. When one feels hungry, s/he can eat but with restricted amount. In real life, most of the patient choose the fast solution, as it is quicker to adjust the body but the side effects are more significant (relatively speaking, slow version has more moderate effects, but they last longer). The side effects include symptoms such as dizziness, headache, back pain, joint pain, palpitation, runny nose, cough, diarrhoea, nausea, itchy skin, etc., resulting in some people giving up halfway.

We have tried two solutions: one is communication, first is to inform them in advance (this is the key): 'while implementing this scheme, most of the people will come across side effects in the initial stage, often, the side effects are the responses to the illness itself. This is normal and suggests positive improvements of the illness, although the process might be painful, the body will be improved after going through this process.' In addition, during the reaction, we try to make the patients confident, and at the same time give professional guidance: either to continue the quick solution or change to slow solution; if the side effects are too strong or influence life and work greatly, it is advisable to stop the treatment temporarily.

The other is the physical therapy, the use of some Chinese medicine, such as acupuncture, cupping, bloodletting, blooding, fire therapy, scraping, etc., to speed up the dredging meridians and relieve symptoms.

Although the two methods mentioned above are effective, the significant side effects are the limitations of the fast solution, and cannot be eliminated completely.

3. Application: As during the tracking and guiding process, the coach does not fully operate the essence of 'educate the patient' scheme, which causes patients to give up halfway or bounce back after adjustment. Although the power of the scheme will make the patients to confirm the significant results and raise the initiative of continuous implementation, the importance of the coach is not ignorable. If the coach does not fully understand the scheme, there will be two kinds of failure during message delivery: one is that patients, who are not great with ignoring interventions and distractions from the environment, will stop because their families do not understand or even, they may oppose the scheme; or they may give up halfway because of the questions and denials from the doctors. The other reason is that the long-term plan is not implemented, but only the 42-day short term plan is focused. This does not help the patients to rebuilt lifestyle, which leads to weigh regain and the relapses of high blood pressure, high blood lipids, and high blood sugar. To avoid the application failure, we have three steps to train the coaches: first, the coaches must have firsthand experience; second, new coaches should consult the experienced coaches; third, the coaches should keep the Coach Manual in mind. Among these, the Coach Manual is the most important. The Coach Manual has been revised seven times, from the first edition of the 18 common questions to the seventh edition with 177 comprehensive and systematic questions; from the initial simple 'question and answer', to the present integration of the mentality and process. This manual has become a professional tool book. Although we have done the above steps to train the coaches, each individual (coach) is different, there are some uncertainties in the results.

In order to reduce dependence on coaches, and reduce the constraints on the development of the career (due to the expansion of the number of coaches and the increase in skills), we have developed two additional educational tools: educational materials and training camps.

Educational information mainly includes educational manuals and educational videos. The contents of the two are basically the same. They explain the causes of lifestyle illness and the ways to solve the problem, the purpose is to deepen the patient's understanding of the method and strengthen the initiative to implement the program. This book can also play the role of education manual. For different groups of people, it can also be abridged into different types of simple version.

The training camp is a comprehensive form of education that we have explored through experimentations. The training camp was formerly a health course. Initially, when we realized the importance of education, it was natural to think of classes for lifestyle groups, including classes for dietary nutrition, sports and psychology, and cultivation of health in different seasons. Yet, later, we found that the efficiency of curriculum education is very low. We spoke a lot, but the patients barely absorbed any knowledge. The implementation of education was also full of mistakes. After 2010, we began to think, could we let the students experience every single lifestyle during class time? This kind of practical counselling allows the students to experience a lifestyle we have been advocating, but we also accompany the students to guide them.

Since 2010, we have changed the training course to training camp that no one had ever seen before. The first time was for 7 days in Chengdu, it was very successful. Every student was convinced because of systematic learning and was excited because of the visible change in body every day. After 7 days, everyone went home, determined to implement the program, and was very clear about how to implement the program. Later, we changed to 5 days camp, and then to 3 days camp, but the low participation rate always confused us. Although those who participated in the training camp could successfully implement the entire program, the number of participants was not a lot, and sometimes dozens of people were planning to participate, but only a few people turned up at the lessons. Therefore, at each training camp, we gave the student a 'feedback sheet', hoping to use the wisdom of the masses to speed up our self-improvement. There was a suggestion to start weekend camps, so that the majority of office workers did not need to ask for a leave and could use the weekend to participate in such experience, which ensured the number of participants. Based on this proposal, we held an intense discussion, the focus of discussion was that only one and a half days of training camp (start on Saturday morning start, end on Sunday noon), could only allow some effects to appear, which may not be enough to let the students to make a decision of whether to participate and complete the program or not. At the end of the discussion, we arrived at a conclusion, we decided to try, and very luckily, we succeeded. The training camp has become our most important means of education ever since. A day and a half days of the training camp has not only solved the problem of low participation rate, but also has maintained a high success rate, of which more than 90% of the students, because of training camp education, are able to eliminate all kinds of interruptions during the process of implement alone, and fully implement short-term programs after the camp. As the team grows, we have found that the training camp can be easily replicated and that a new coach with certain knowledge can organize a new training camp after participating on one or two courses, so we have grown from the initial one session a month to multiple per month. The numbers of participants vary from a few people to hundreds, the most ideal is thirty or fifty people. We also tried half a day experience camp. The participants learn for half a day, and take the food with them as they leave the camp. They come back the next morning to measure changes in indexes, then eat breakfast. The effects are also very good.

We have tried many different the contents for the training camp, including group discussions, speeches, examinations and replies, scoring and awards, and even evening entertainment parties. These are all effective interactions, and can be arranged flexibly according to the context. We think the three basic contents are: lectures, sharing and experiencing, among them the most important is experiencing. There have been some fixed standard classes for lectures; sharing is to ask the experienced learners to share their experiences. Experiencing is to practice the case in real, including catering, snacks, sports, drinking water and so on.

One-to-one counselling, educational materials and training camps, these three kinds of educational means should complement each other. Professional coaches can carry out one-to-one education, but cannot ignore the use of auxiliary tools. Human capacity is limited, but the application of the tool is infinite. Videos are suitable for those who have convenient access to Internet; an hour of scientific educational videos have good effects. Books are more suitable for higher-quality people, especially professional doctors. Reading allows an in-depth and long-lasting self-education. One of the major purposes of this book is to promote basic education, but it still cannot completely replace the training camp. Experiencing, as the core of the training camp, is an important means of behaviour training. However, even if the training camp is comprehensive and thorough, we still need one-to-one education, which include explanation before the camp and check-ups after training camp.

Although the efforts and work (as mentioned above) cannot completely eliminate failures during actual practice, the purpose is more and more apparent – focus on education. Focus on training both the coaches and the patients, educate the mind and the behaviour at the same time. With the deepening of research work, the above work has yet to be improved, and even further, we need to create better methods. Yet, no matter what kind of method, if they are classified by 'who will implement the method', it can be divided into three categories: first and foremost is self-education; followed by education by patients (sharing of experiences); then education from experts. Evaluation of the effectiveness of education has two basic indicators: first, whether the metabolic issues, such as high blood pressure, high blood sugar, hyperlipidaemia and obesity have been improved in the short term. Second, whether the correct habits have been established, and whether the simple but effective method have been mastered, in a long-term view.

Chapter One: Practical Case

This book has chosen some common representative cases from the success (most cases are successful cases. The purpose is not to make a final academic summary, as experiments are still being carried out extensively, and the relevant data and statistics are accumulating. The purpose of selecting the following cases is to discuss specific issues with real-life examples to better illustrate the theory presented in this book. Basically, each case represents a type (of issues and patients) encountered in practice, which together represents the summary of our ten years of practice. If the reader has a different view of the analysis on the specific case, you are welcome to give feedback to us (luboshishu@163.com), and we feel grateful for your kind comments.

In order to make finding the contents you are interested in easier, we have divided the cases into obesity category and disease category, but in fact it is often difficult to completely separate them. The best thing we can do is that for some cases we focus on obesity more, while for some cases, we mainly discuss the disease. Because of the large number of test results, and they do not have a unified form, in order to keep it succinct, we only provide some cases to represent the whole group, these cases are for reference only.

Here we would like to express our thanks to all the students who have selflessly provides their changes and true feelings to the public, and to encourage others to become healthy earlier. Each case is written by the patients themselves, although they may differ in style, but they are all good stories with true feelings. Each person shares their own experience, and make a unique contribution to the world in their own way. Here, I would like to pay a deep tribute to them!

Disease

Case 1:

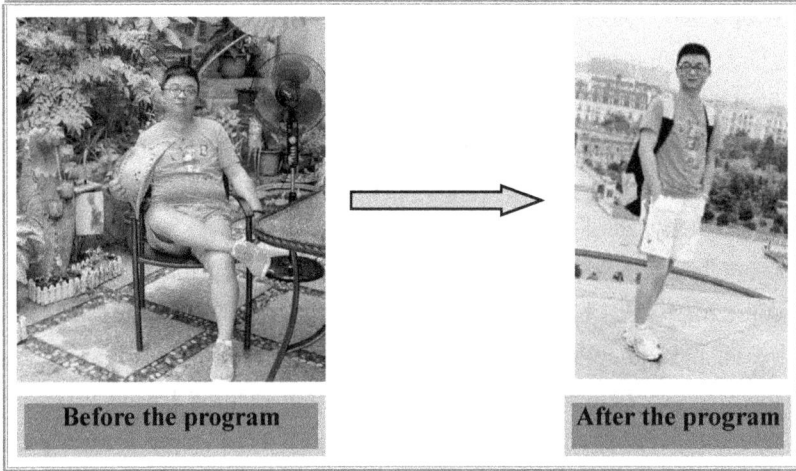

| | Before the program | After the program |

My name is Yong Ding. I come from Hangzhou, below is my physical data before and after I took part in Doctor Lu's program:

	Before program	After program
Weight	81.5kg	65kg (two cycles)
BMI	28.9	23
Waistline	103cm	82cm
Blood uric acid	417μmol/L	280μmol/L
Triglycerides	7.77μmol/L	1.21μmol/L
Total cholesterol	6.40μmol/L	5.37μmol/L
Fatty liver	moderate	N/A

Let me tell you about my adjustment experience. My parents are retired old military doctors, so I can be said to be born in a medical family. I was obese and had been used to it for years. Whereas my parents were very anxious when watching my belly which made me look like I was pregnant for 6-7 months. They kept telling me that I was so fat, the body would certainly have a lot of problems, and it was time for me to lose weight, eat less, and do more exercise. After listening to their words, I always smiled. For obesity, I was not in a hurry. In my own opinion, obesity was nothing more than just more fat in thebody than other people, and my life was not different when compared with normal people, so I never thought about losing weight. Don't laugh at me, in 2007, when a colleague of mine who was pregnant, and went to work with her pregnant belly. During that time, I often compared the abdominal width with her, and I was very proud, that others are only pregnant for ten months, I was pregnant for ten years. We also contested who had the bigger belly, and I won by 103cm to 96cm.

Under the constant urge from my parents, and I forced myself to try some methods. I had been working in healthcare product industry for 20 years, and I knew well about the sneaky tricks of this industry, so I never touched any healthcare products. The main method I used was to eat less and exercise more like my parents said. After doing it for a period of time, I bore a lot of pressure, but the weight change was not obvious, and when the weather was not good, I could not exercise. I did not have any more courage of carrying on and I had given up finally. I still lived calmly with my fat body, and never thought about losing weight again.

What really woke me up was a physical examination organized by my company. In the blood Comprehensive Metabolic Panel results, there was a row of a rising arrows, and it shook me. This time, I began to worry. With so many indicators that did not meet the standards, how was I going to do? The inconvenience of obesity suddenly came to my heart. Yet, it is quite difficult to find the most suitable one among all those healthcare methods.

Later, on the recommendation of a friend, I participated in Dr. Lu's program. Initially I was also dubious, but for the sake of health, I still asked myself to listen to the coach. In the 42-day short-term plan, I strictly performed the requirements given by the coach, and ate fish, meat, tofu and vegetables every day, and stayed away from the staple food. I walked to digest after dinner every day. I lost 10kg by the 28th day of the program. What was amazing was that the snoring situation also disappeared during sleep. This was really a surprise. It was no exaggeration to say that my snoring was sometimes louder than a train, which affected those who were next to me in the train! My colleagues who went on business trips with me were very painful from the snoring, and wished to stay away from me as far as possible. Curiosity drove me to the hospital to do a Comprehensive Metabolic Panel after participating in the program, except for moderate fatty liver, all the other arrows miraculously disappeared. I took the inspection report home to show to my parents, and they looked at me with a very strange look and said, 'It is not possible. It is certainly a mistake made by the nurse.' I also had such kind of doubts after listening to what they said; after all, they had been acting as army doctors for their life.

However, a doubt was only a doubt. Everybody witnessed how I had lost some weight, and as always, I did according to the requirements of the coach and finished the next two weeks of adjustment. Throughout the cycle, my weight dropped by 11.5kg. In order to verify the physical examination results during adjustment, I went to the hospital again to do the Comprehensive Metabolic Panel and B ultrasound, and the results were the same with the previous ones, all indicators were back to normal, fatty liver also disappeared! By then, I no longer doubted the magic of Dr. Lu's program. I excitedly took the inspection report back home, my parents were also convinced. Yet, as to my adjustment results, the father is still more worried, he said to me that fast weight loss would do harm to your body. To answer his queries again, I said that now the fact was that I had lost weight, and that it was also true that my indicators were back to normal, meanwhile my mental state was better than ever before. There was nothing that can speak more than truth.

Under the guidance of confidence, I followed the second cycle of adjustment strictly. It felt easy and relaxed as always, and I lost 5kg. After two cycles, I reached the target of losing 16.5 kg, which made me very happy and pleased. Dr. Lu's solution has solved my fatty liver which had accompanied me for many years, it has made my blood indicators back to normal, and I finally have neck again (before when I was fat, everybody said that I didn't have neck because it was covered by fat); what's more is that the layers on my stomach, which had been with me for years, also have disappeared. It has been 3 years since I completed the cycles. Now my weight maintains below 67.5kg, and I feel relaxed, I sleep well and have a high spirit, and also have kept away from the 'rich man's disease'. Now I have become one of the advocates of the program. I join them, and put in all efforts to do it, hoping that more and more people can understand and benefit from it earlier.

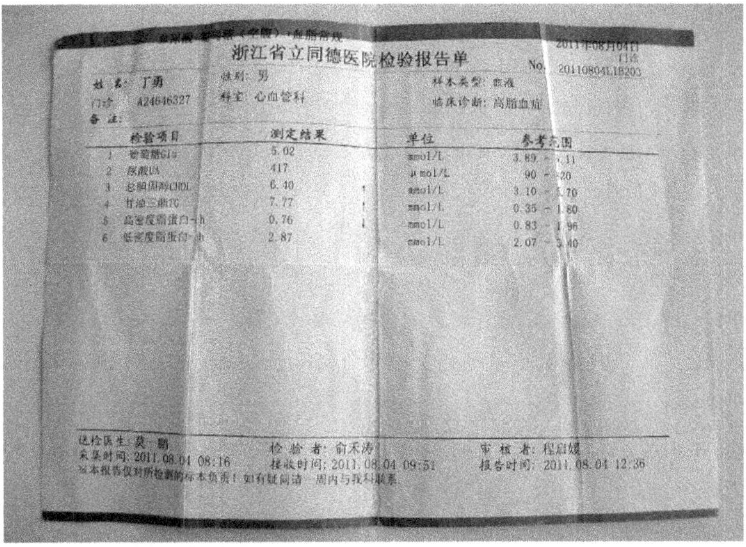

Before the program

After the program

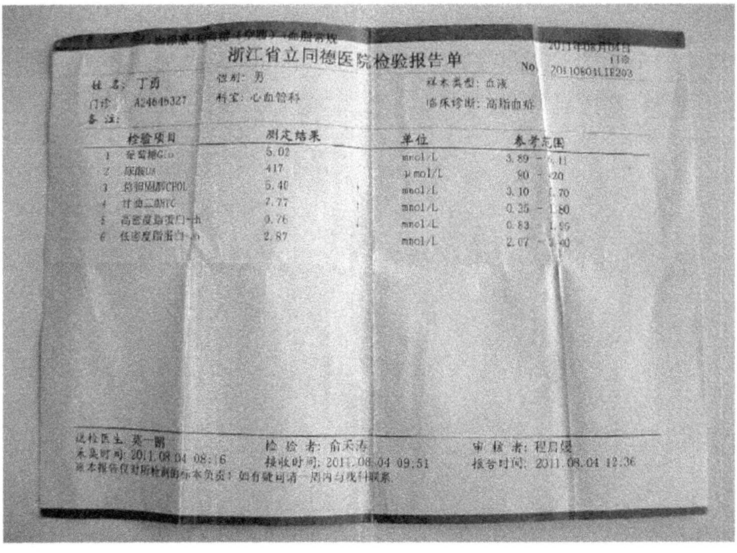

Comments:

As a military doctor, Mr. Ding's parents did not believe in the effects which the program has achieved at the end of the first cycle, which was very common. Doctors with theoretical knowledge and actual experience are sceptical about the effect. This experience also deeply affected hundreds of millions of patients. Triple H patients, almost with no exception, are informed by doctors that this is a lifelong disease, and it is necessary to take drugs for life. The outdated belief constraints people's minds. When the truth arises, most people doubt it, or even ridicule it, which is perhaps the norm of history. 200 years ago, when Watt invented the steam engine and started the human industrial revolution; the British newspaper also ridiculed it like this: 'if the steam can drive the train to run, a person can go to heaven by putting a fart!' If one thing is true, but most people do not believe it, what does it mean? The reason is that the thing is too good to be true. Yet, if it is in fact true, the doubts must be temporary. It is always that a small part of the people firstly grasp the truth, which leads to more people to know the truths, and then the truth becomes common sense. It fulfils the phrase 'truth is often in the hands of a few people.' Therefore, the spread of truth takes time.

Case 2:

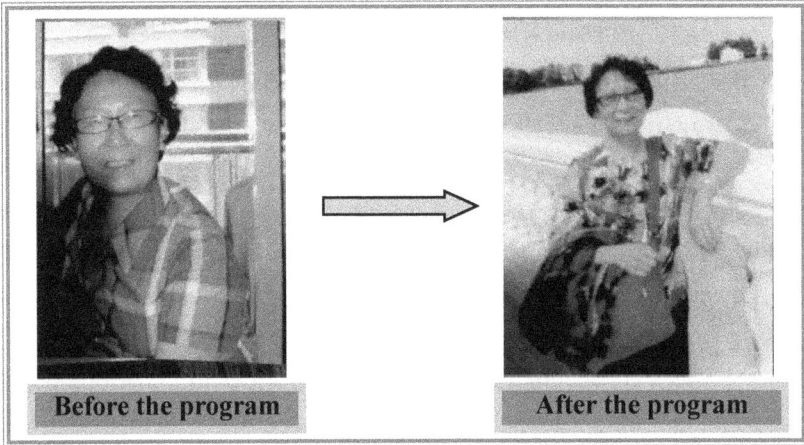

| Before the program | After the program |

My name is Fang Hou, and I was born in April 1940, aged 74, a retired teacher.

In July 2011, I heard one of my friend said that there was a method that could cure Triple H, and I was interested in it.

When I gave birth to my child at the age of 23, the doctor shouted outside of the delivery room that: 'relatives of the maternal, do not leave; the blood pressure of the mother is too high!' After that, my blood pressure had been unstable. However, I did not feel anything, and knew little about it, paid no attention to it because I was young and immature. The pressures from life and work became heavier and heavier with age, my body gradually became weak. I graduated from college in 1962, and I worked as a high school math teacher for years, especially the senior class and acted as Main Teacher (in China, the main teacher teaches while also takes care of the class from every different aspect, while other teachers only teach) at the same time. I worked every day busily, from dawn to dusk with the students who were going to take college entrance examination. As a result, my blood pressure problem became more and more severe, and I had to take pills. I started going to the hospital to seea doctor and get medicine. The medicine changed again and again, and I ate more and more. Although the pressure reduced after retirement, but the blood pressure was not taking a turn for the better.

In July 2011 before the adjustment, my daily dosage was: half tablet of Bose 5 mg, one Amlodipine Besylate Tablets, one 0.15g Irbesartan, and sometimes needed to add one more. Even such, it could not be controlled sometimes. Sometimes in the evening, my blood pressure would reach up to 180/75-85, and needed additional pills. Yet, every drug had certain toxicity. While inhibiting the disease, side effects also followed. I was very distressed when looking at the table with a row of tablet bottles on it.

I was 1.57 meters high, weighed 57.5 kg at time. In this case, I thought that weight loss is not important, I would try any method as long as my blood pressure could be cured, and the method would allow me to reduce my dosage of medicine.

July 2011, my friend and I participated in the training camp. In the lecturers, we thought the lectures and experts had a valid point and seemed reasonable. Then we started the program, we strictly followed every requirement as asked by the program. After one cycle of 42 days, the effects were obviously visible.

First, the dosage of drugs was gradually reduced in the adjustment process. If I didn't reduce the dosage, the blood pressure would very low, and sometimes only reached 90. The least amount drug intake was only half tablet of Amlodipine Besylate a day. Blood pressure was generally stable at 120/70. Until now two years later, I only take half tablet of antihypertensive drug a day, and add to one tablet when it is too cold in winter.

Second, I felt like that this method was safe and effective regarding losing weight. I lost 5 kg, now my weight is less than 52.5kg. I feel better than before and full of spirit. At present, I can take 4 classes with dozens of people in in the classes; I can drive alone to the suburbs, Tianjin and other places with energetic spirit and stable blood pressure.

I am very satisfied because the adjustment not only reduced the number of medication I took, but also stabilized blood pressure. Through the lessons in the adjustment program, I have learned about the right lifestyle, balanced diets, and daily exercise. I also often share my experience with my friends, guide them to know about the decent program, and wish them to have a healthy and happy life.

Comments:

The implementation of the program included drug withdrawal and drug reduction. According to the laws and patterns, elderlies with long history of sickness can reduce drug usage, but sometimes cannot achieve complete withdrawal. We have found that this is related to the degree of organ damages, as well as the tissues' renewable capacity, the stronger the renewable capacity, the more likely the full recovery. If the regeneration capacity is weak, the possibility of complete recovery is low; the part of the drug reduced is the part that the body can recover.

Case 3:

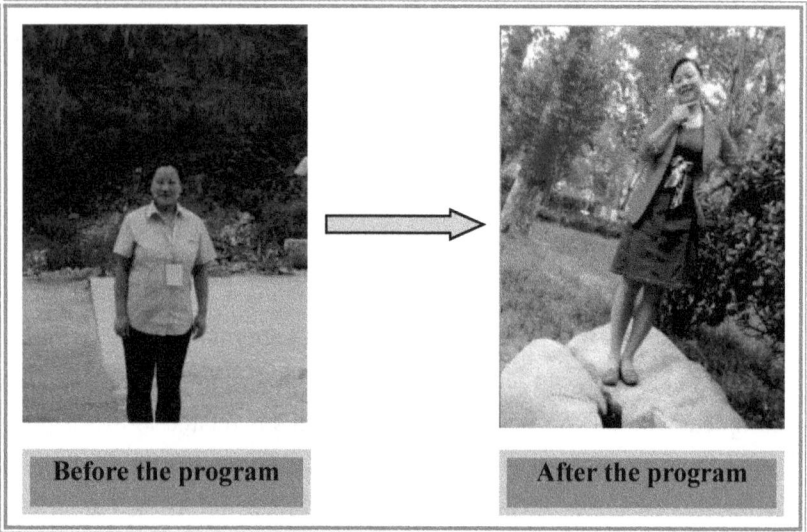

Before the program   After the program

Yunhong Zhu, female, 35 years old, a program promoter.

Many mothers were worried that weight would gain after giving births, and so did I. After giving birth, my weight rapidly grew to 71.5kg. My main concern was that my stomach did not recover well, and I looked like I was seven or eight months into pregnancy. Every time I took bus, the warm-hearted ticket seller gave me her seat. The embarrassment was more than a thankful heart, but I also had to explain that I was not pregnant. In 2009 my son was born with the weight of 4.9 kg. Because he was a big baby, I was included in the 'high risk of diabetes' group. This was confirmed when my son is 2 years old, I became a diabetic. In addition to my increasing weight, a lot of sub-health signals appeared in my body: dizziness, chest tightness, irritability and slow actions. I felt like that I suddenly became old. At that time, I once suspected that I had gotten some diseases. After checking at the hospital, the results showed that my blood glucose was as high as 7.3, which meant that I was a diabetes patient. I felt down as I was so young when I got such kind of disease.

Perhaps God blessed me, and let me know about Dr. Lu's program. After one cycle of treatment, my weight reduced from 71.5kg to 59kg, a total reduction of 12.5kg. Although I still have not met my ideal weight I wanted, compared with the previous, I have been contented. Blood sugar also has returned to normal - 5.8, and my big belly also magically disappeared. All kinds of sub-health signals are gone, and I have become more confident and cheerful. I do not need to buy clothes in the exclusive store for overweight people anymore.

What was unexpected was that allergic rhinitis that had troubled me for many years also disappeared. I was very sensitive to the smell of cigarettes before. Whenever I smelled it, my nose would immediately become intolerably itchy like my nose had numerous insects moving it. When it was serious, it bled every morning, and my breathing was not smooth, which was very painful. After the adjustment, one day, I was waiting for the bus, someone next to me was smoking, I moved unconsciously, but the smells of cigarettes also moved with me. However, this time, my nose did not itch, but just smelled the cigarette, I was so excited and felt like crying. For a long time, I always worried about the relapse of rhinitis. However, it has been one year since the program, I can still breathe smoothly, and the allergic rhinitis that had tortured me for years had finally gone. Yeah!!!

Since I am the beneficiary of this program, I hope that more friends who are troubled by metabolic diseases can benefit from it like how I did. With confidence and responsibilities, I have become a promoter of this program. For more than a year, I do my best to help a lot of friends, and make them indicators normal again from an overweight and unhealthy state. I am grateful and proud to see their affirmations to the program. I thank the developers for their wisdom and mind, I am proud to have this method, there is no doubt that I am lucky to have such program. Meanwhile I believe that I can make more people get health and have a happy family.

Comments:

Allergic rhinitis is very difficult to cure with both Chinese medicine and Western Medicine. Why? Because what it presents is the complex health problem inside the body. Nasal methods do not often achieve good results when treating rhinitis. Some people say that lungs connect with the nose, so we should adjust the lung. Yet the lungs connect with intestines, the health of the intestines determines the health of the lungs. So, the problem cannot be solved by simply treating the lungs. It also has direct relationships with the immune system. When the immune system is weak, the respiratory system is vulnerable to external environment, which results in asthma, influenza, and allergic rhinitis. So it is a complex physical problem. For such complex physical problems, the solution is to adjust the whole body. Under the case of whole-body adjustment, problems of some parts of the body can easily be improved, but this systemic problem reflects through a certain part of the body. It would be difficult to cure the problem if we only dealt with the part, or the organ that associated with that part that manifested the problem. Our method differs from other methods in that it is a set of systemic adjustments. It is not medicine that fights against rhinitis, nor an enhancement for an organ, but it is the overall adjustment of the body. For example, the improvement of immune system, the adjustment of intestinal flora and the filling of lung, addition of these makes the body healthy again, weight loss is also part of the benefits of the body.

Case 4:

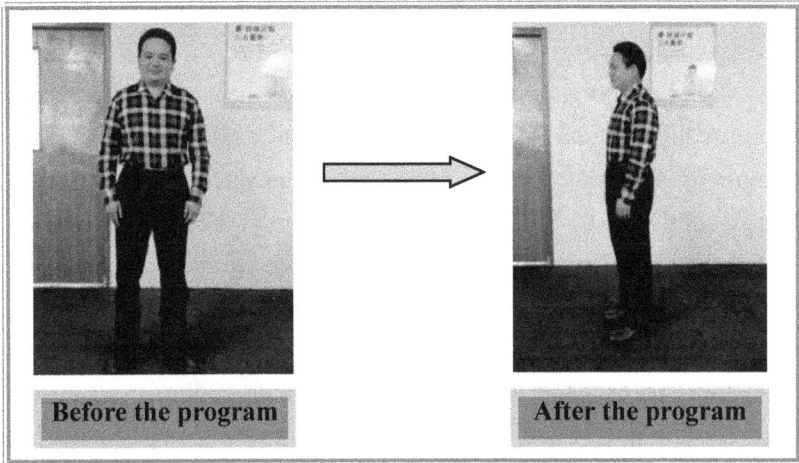

Before the program → After the program

My name is Jinjian Wu, 36 years old, 168cm height, from the Hunan Province. Below are my measurements and statistics before and after I took part in Doctor Lu's adjustment scheme.

Item	Before program	Before program
Weight	90 Kg	70Kg (two cycles)
BMI	31.8	24.8
Waistline	110cm	83cm
Triglycerides	6.53μmol/L	0.82μmol/L
Total cholesterol	7.40μmol/L	4.36μmol/L
Fatty liver	moderate	N/A

I have been in health management for a full decade. As Deputy Secretary General of the Hunan Provincial Health Management Institute, my main job is to study the business model of health management industry and health management service to promote the development of Hunan health management industry. With the responsibility and enthusiasm for this industry, in the past decade, I have travelled almost all over China, and have visited a lot of industries and projects related to health management. Meanwhile given that the current health management market in Hunan is limited to only healthy physical examination, and the service after examination has not been put into practice, I hope to seek some good ways to make up for the lack of follow-up service market, and lead the provincial health examination to a deeper level in health management field.

I had also regretted, because as a health management worker, and one of the members of health management experts' team in Hunan, my body was out of shape. At the annual physical examinations, my triglycerides and total cholesterol went beyond the average, and I had moderate fatty liver. When I stood on the podium and shared health management related knowledge with my students, the participants often told me jokingly: 'Mr Wu, your sharing of health management services course is really good, but as you stand on the podium, you look like a typical Triple H and obese patient! If you are going to teach more detailed healthy management knowledge, it is less persuasive.' Every time, after listening to what they said, I felt ashamed. Of course, as a healthy management worker, I knew clearly the dangers of Triple H and obesity. I had tried a lot of methods, such as controlling food intake and exercise, but every time it ended up with failures because I liked meat and disliked exercising.

I should thank one of my bosses in Health Department who specially introduced me to this method, so that I could know about Doctor Lu's Scheme. After preliminary understanding, I thought that the theoretical basis of this method was consistent with the concept of modern medicine and the theoretical principles of health management. It was a combination of clinical medicine, preventive medicine, Chinese medicine, health management, nutrition, psychology, and kinematics. After less than a month, in August 2012, I immediately took my team to Beijing to study, and participated in the training camp. In a relaxed and happy environment, the results of the next day, after I had experienced for one day, really shook me. My weight reduced by 1.2 kg, not only me, but also almost all members of our team lost weight. What excited me was that I could lose weight even if I ate meat. In addition, this method did not need medicine, injections, health care products and medical equipment. Only lifestyle management was needed to solve the diabetes, which even the clinical medicine could not solve. I thought it was really amazing. So, I made a bold decision to bring this technology back to Hunan. One is considering the broad prospects for the application of this technology. It can be used as an intervention technology after inspection in medical centre to make up for the market blank of post-intervention. Also, the technical operation is convenient, simple, effective, and easy to be implemented by an individual. It can be carried out in a large area to lead the provincial health examination to a deeper level in health management field, and bring benefits for the people in Hunan; second is considering that the technology can be used as a practical skill for the vocational skills training of health management experts, in order to enhance the power of our health management division team; third is considering my own obesity.

Of course, when a new technology is to be promoted in a new area, it must establish a model. Without experiments, the proposal is weak. I followed the coach's guidance, and fully experienced two cycles of short-term plans, and verified the effectiveness of the method by my practical acting. For 84 days, my weight decreased by 20 kg, the size of my waist drop from the original 3.3 feet to 2.5 feet, and round belly disappeared. What pleased me more was that my original abnormal metabolic indicators were normal, B ultrasonic showed that moderate fatty liver, that had accompanied me for years, had miraculously disappeared. Before I always snored ask loud as thunders, and sometimes I had sleep apnoea symptom. Now the degree of snoring has reduced and I am more energetic. When standing on the podium, I am no longer afraid of the jokes of the students about I am a typical Triple H and obese patient, which is kind of relief. It has been two years after finishing the intervention, my weight has been kept well because I have changed my old bad habits, and established the correct way of life. I eat more coarse grains and less refined grains, I exercise every day, insist on taking trace elements to ensure the balance of metabolism.

Now our team is constantly growing, I will spare no effort to contribute more, and share the results of this program to more friends, so that more people can get rid of obesity and Triple H as soon as possible.

Comments:

Like Secretary Wu, many people marvel at the miraculous effects of this program. Nevertheless, we must emphasize that, it is not the magic of the program but magic of instinct. External causes can only work through internal factors. The program focuses on how to stimulate people's life potentials, how to maximize the human self-healing instinct, how to restore the body's inherent metabolism of blood pressure, blood sugar, blood lipid, to achieve drug reduction or even drug withdrawal. We believe that this is the right direction of medical science. The medical miracles cannot be made without instinctive support.

Case 5:

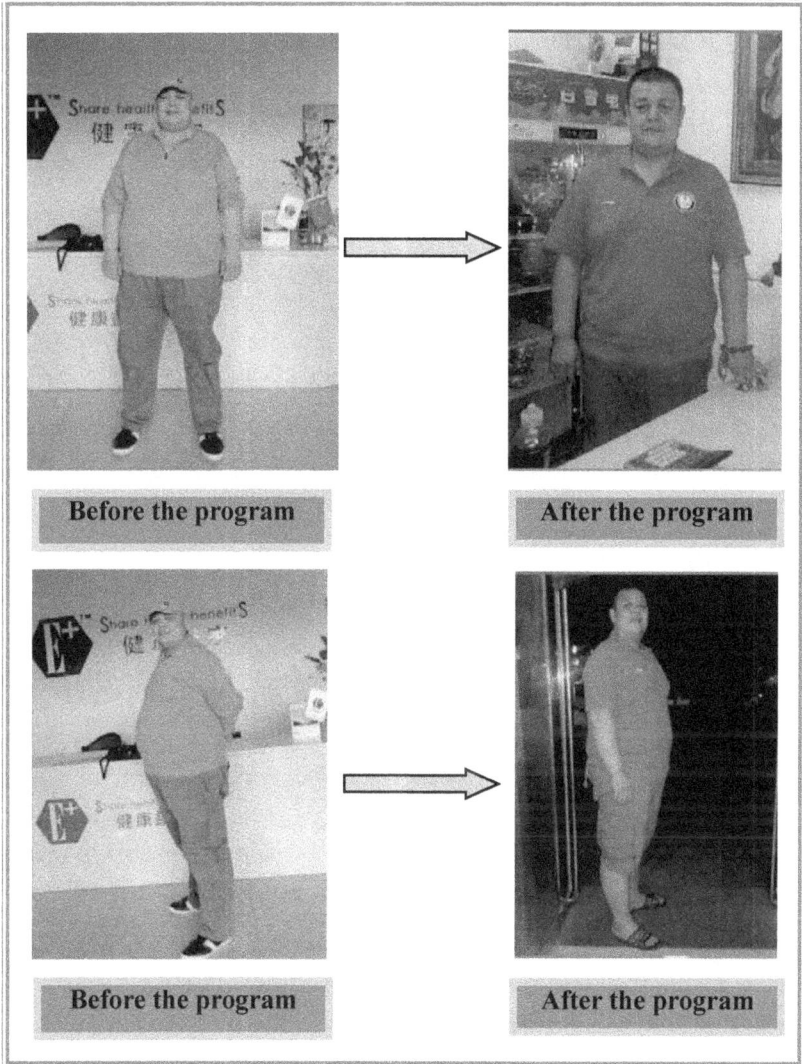

My name is Zhigang Liu (father of Hongyu Liu, from obesity category, case 3), born in Heilongjiang Province on 21st June 1971. I was the youngest child at home, because I was spoilt by my parents, I had developed a bad habit of eating irregularly. In everyone's eyes, I was a little fat child, as time went by I gradually grew into a big fat man.

I am responsible for the sale of the company. In such a working environment; I need to invite customers over for dinner. I always overate, and my weight jumped up to be over 100 kg from the original 90kg when I first started my career. After marriage, with the birth of my child I started my own business; both my marriage and career were very stable. Because of the type of my work, I dined with customers outside every day, and wine became my best friend. I had dinner dates with friends and customers every day. A few years later, my body collapsed. The hospital diagnosed me with diabetes, pre-meal blood sugar was 14.7, and postprandial blood sugar was 23.1. After that, I started on the long journey of treating the disease and began to take hypoglycemic drugs called Metformin for nearly two years. This medicine had great side effects: irritated kidneys, back pain, limbs weakness, and urine difficulty. I visited the doctor and he changed to an imported drug called Repaglinide with fewer side effects. I took this medicine for more than three years, started from half pill to one pill and then one and a half pill. Although with fewer side effects, it was often said that any drug has toxicity, and the longer time I took the medicine for, the weaker the effects of the medicine on the disease. I often heard people talking that diabetes was like an immortal cancer, and this really stressed me. When I had nothing to do, I thought about how I would not be able to recover, and how I had to spend the rest of my life with diabetes. I felt desperate when I thought of this.

At the beginning of 2012, my wife discussed with me regarding the future of my kid. She said she want to ask him to join the army. I was in a mood of crying and laughing; my kid had the same body shape as me, and it would be a joke if he was going to join the army. My son is Hongyu Liu, might be because of the eating habits of our family, he reached 150kg in weight. As soon as he reached 18 years old, he dropped from school and stayed at home, his future had become an unsolvable problem in the household. My son once dreamed of joining the army, but it was totally impossible based on the current situation (one must not be overweight to join the army). Yet, my wife was very persistent, and seeking all kinds of methods to help us to lose weight. By chance, she got to know Doctor Lu's scheme, and after many times of detailed consulting, the coach had designed a whole set of adjustment plan for my son: meal adjustment and exercise plan. Starting from May, 2012, my wife and son started to meddle in the weight losing program, but to me, it was ridiculous. The menus read that meat was allowed for nutrition meal, also vegetables and fruits, but no staple food. It was new and differed from the normal ways, but I still did not believe that it would help with weight loss.

As time went by for 3 months, I could not believe my eyes when I saw the changes my son had made day by day. For the first month, he lost more than 20kg, and he had rested for several days without bouncing back. He became diligent and full of vitality. With all kinds of curiosity, I attended a health training camp and listened to the experts to explain the health knowledge, as well as the causes for obesity, diabetes and so on. Seeing the beneficiaries sharing their experiences one after another, especially my son Liu Hongyu, and it was the first time I had seen him so confident when walking up to the stage, speaking with spirit of his experience and planning his future which moved me many times over. I asked myself secretly, even my son had the determination to do it, and I was obese and with diabetes, why couldn't I accompany my son and walk together towards an experience that might change his life forever. Before my son stepped down from the stage, I could not help myself from appearing on the stage next to him, and told him: 'We should battle like father and son in the battle field and compete. I might not understand all your previous hardships, but from today on I will accompany you!'

As it became, the coach developed a special program for me according to my situation. What interested me the most was my blood sugar problem; I did not care about the weight. Because I was at a middle age with a wife and a child, weight was not so important for me. However, my physical condition put me close to the danger of injecting insulin. In the next few months, my son and I encouraged each other and my wife prepared the meal strictly in accordance with the requirements of the menu. After a week, I stopped the hypoglycemic drug taken at noon, and a few days later, I reduced the drugs eaten in morning and evening by half, and for a month, I only relied on taking my hypoglycemic drugs. My weight was constantly decreasing. Because of the needs of business I continued to participate in social events weight loss was not very fast. On the other hand, my child successfully lost 50kg and joined the army at the end.

After my child left for the army, I have stopped all drugs for more than six months now, and my blood sugar is at a normal level. More importantly, I can taste a variety of long-lost seasonal fruits, no longer avoid certain foods. Maybe everyone is surprised that I have lost over 30kg after executing two cycles of short-term program. These are not enough to let me reach the normal weight range. However, two-cycles and nearly three-month adjustment have fundamentally changed our eating habits. The balanced diet, moderate miscellaneous grains and less refined staple food effectively help to control my blood sugar.

Thanks to Dr. Lu program, every family member now has a healthy body. Every time I see those who are suffering from Triple H, I really fear that they will repeat my mistakes and can't help but to share with them my weight loss process. I sincerely hope that more diabetes patients like me can get to know Dr. Lu's program earlier to get rid of the pain.

Comments:

The establishment of lifestyle should be based on a family. Diabetes often occurs by family unit, so many people mistakenly believe that it is genetic. In fact, it is not genetic inheritance, but 'genetic' by the way of lifestyle. Our intervention is not from one person to another, but from one family to another one, to establish a correct way of lifestyle, so as to establish a healthy family culture. This culture will be handed down generation to generation. It will not only change a family, but also a nation. Our experiments have proved that it is not only feasible to use lifestyle to solve lifestyle disease, but also this method is the most cost efficient, the best and longest lasting.

Case 6:

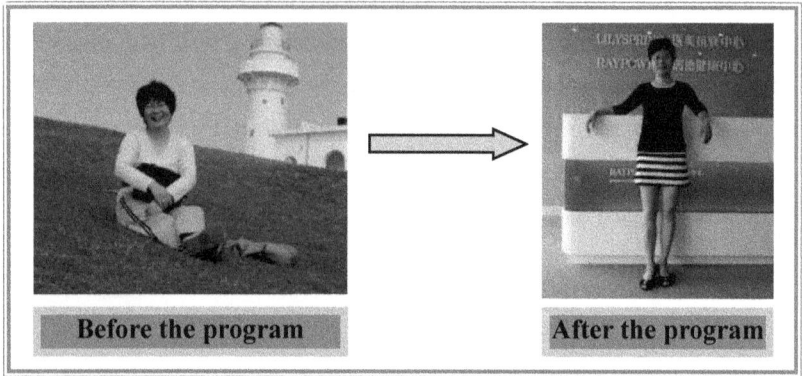

| Before the program | After the program |

I am Mei Wu (sister of Jing Wu from obesity category case 7), born in 1962. When my mother was pregnant with me, she worked at the Chinghai Water Conservancy Site. The condition was harsh, only cabbage was available. After I was born, my mother had mastitis, and she fed me while injecting streptomycin. I was fed like this for two months, them my mother went back to Chinghai again. I was raised up by my grandmother with a small amount of milk and rice soup, so my body conditions was not good since an early age. I was misdiagnosed with arthritis at college, and was treated with a lot of penicillin and hormones. However, my joints didn't get better and my health deteriorated. After that, I had all kinds of suboptimal health symptoms: headache, stomach pain, diarrhoea, chest tightness, shortness of breath, back pain, fatigue, upset, poor sleep, easy to dream, easy to wake up, hard to fall asleep, difficult to concentrate and such. For decades, I relied on Traditional Chinese Medicine and acupuncture treatment. Sometimes the conditions are good, but sometimes terrible. My menstruation went out of order when I was 42 years old, the menopause was even worse. I gained more than 15 kg, and the symptoms became more and more severe. I constantly got new diseases, I could not climb stairs due to joint pain, I could not do anything and struggled to live by myself. I felt like life was meaningless at the age of 50.

Participation in the camp was unplanned, but it changed me. Encouraged by the coach, I ate apples and eggs that I dared not before (before, I would have stomach discomfort and diarrhoea, etc. after eating them.). Yet, the next day, not only that there was or discomfort, my eyes also were brighter. These were unexpected. This attempt greatly encouraged me, so I was determined to change and adjust my lifestyle. After 42-day short-term plan, I was like a new person. Not only that I lost 7.5kg, but also all old problems, like sleep difficulty, stomach, swollen and headache, disappeared. In addition, my mental and physical strength increased, sleeping quality was better, the vitality was doubled, it felt refreshing from hand to toe, and I felt much younger. Now I am in love with this program because it keeps people healthy and keep them away from sickness. Also it helps people to perform new and correct lifestyles in everyday life, and the whole family is also involved.

Comments:

Ms. Wu's is a typical case where the patient has taken large number of drugs for many years, including Traditional Chinese Medicine and Western Medicine. The program does not use medication, but the effects are better than that treatments with Traditional Chinese Medicine or Western Medicine, this fully shows that treatment based on changes in diet is better than medical therapy. The program is a combination of diet treatment (Traditional Chinese Medicine) and nutrition balance (Western Medicine), meanwhile important innovation is made in methods. The core idea of the method is the energy conversion theory (turning waste into wealth). Therefore, the effects are not only better than Traditional Chinese Medicine and Western Medicine, but even better than diet treatment of Traditional Chinese Medicine and nutrition balance of Western Medicine. The key is that energy conversion exploits human instinct to a great extent.

Case 7:

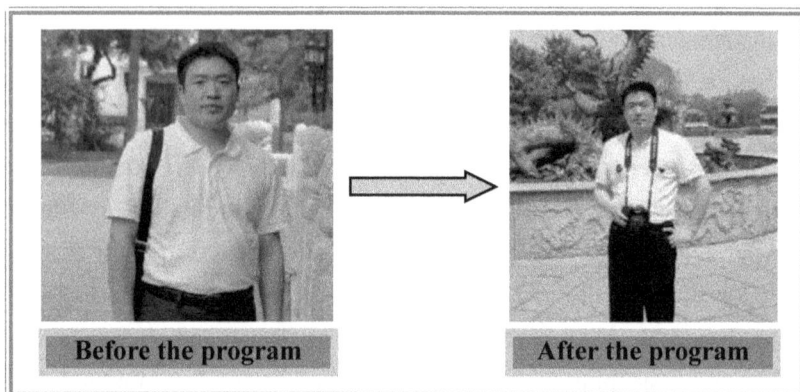

| Before the program | After the program |

My name is Jian Wu (husband of Ying Wen, from obesity category case 4) (father of Chianlingfang Wu, from obesity category case 4) from Guiyang, 45 years old, have now settled in Beijing. Below is my data before and after I attended the Dr. Lu program:

	Before program	After program
Weight	72.5kg	61.5kg
Waistline	93.33cm	83.33cm
Blood pressure	110/115	82/120
Left knee joint	Sever pain, difficulty in walking	Pain relieved, walk normally

The change was something I never dared to imagine, and I never dared to expect to happen, because my way to seek medical treatment can be described as with hardships. This course let me full of hope sometime, but sometimes makes me extremely hopeless!

China's greatest literary theorist, Mr. Guowei Wang, in his classic 'Human Words', described the three realms of those who wanted to achieve something great, my medical treatment journey was exactly the same with Mr. Wang's three realms. Now when I look back, I am filled with a thousand kinds of emotions!

I used to work in the media industry, including magazines, newspapers and websites, and worked for nearly ten years. During that time, I started from journalist to editor, editor to chief editor, and then to president. With the promotion of title, I worked overtime more and more. Very often, in order to catch up with a news article that needed to be written immediately, I often worked until late at night while others were asleep. It was common to eat midnight snacks and drink a little beer to lighten up my spirit. From long period of irregular lifestyle and uncontrolled diet, I started to gain weight and suffered from high blood pressure. At first, I did not care much, and always thought that a good rest for some time would be fine. However, things were not as easy as I had imagined, my blood pressure was still high. Every time I went to hospital because of a cold, the doctor was shocked after a test of blood pressure, and then advised me to take antihypertensive drugs as soon as possible. On the other hand, my friends who had high blood pressure advised strongly that I shall not eat antihypertensive drugs easily, saying that it was a temporary solution which could not cure the core issue, and I should try to adjust through Traditional Chinese Medicine or Traditional Chinese Medicine therapy. So, I thought: what kind of Traditional Chinese Medicine and health methods could cure my disease? I began to try to find Chinese medicine remedies and health essence with all my might.

One day, I entered the first realm: 'the west wind withered the tree last night; alone I walked up to the high-raised tower, and looked at the horizon.' In order to reduce blood pressure, I looked for a lot of Chinese Medicine experts, got lots of prescription, and ate a variety of Traditional Chinese Medicine. Some Traditional Chinese Medicine tasted fine, and some smelled obnoxious, and difficult to drink. Yet, for the sake of health, I tried my hardest and swallowed down all kinds of drugs, which could only be described as miserable! However, there were no signs of a decrease blood pressure. What made me more difficult to bear was that starting from the end of 2011, my left knee joint started to hurt. At first I did not take much notice, thinking that it was due to lots of walk and the meridians were hurt, and it would be fine after a rest for a while, but the pain became more and more severe, casing difficulties when walking and squatting. This was even worse for a hypertensive patient like me.

So I went to the best orthopaedic hospital in Beijing- Jishuitan Hospital for treatment, after seeing my knee image taken by the radiology department, a young doctor told me that because of my meniscus damage and collateral ligament injury was never fully recovered, I would feel painful when walking. Finally, the young doctor said: 'Nothing to worry, I will give you some medicine to eat, then all will be fine.' Seeing the confidence in doctor's eyes, I thought I would say farewell to the sick legs soon, I was quite pleased. But my leg pain did not become any better after taking the medicine for three months later. So, from the beginning of 2012 to August 2013, I had to put down the work, travelled around, and sought for medical treatment for my leg and blood pressure. During this period, I not only drank a variety of decoctions of Traditional Chinese Medicine and wiped various kinds of external use Chinese herbal medication, but also tried all kinds of Traditional Chinese Medicine therapy, including fire therapy, acupuncture, cupping, negative oxygen push, fumigation, steam therapy, etc., and bought a variety of expensive health products and a variety of supplements. If anyone claimed that something was useful to reduce blood pressure and joint pains, I was willing to spend money, but the effects were always tiny. In particular, a few days before the Chinese New Year in 2013, a friend said that water spa could eradicate leg pain completely, I believed and let him do the water spa on me, Who would thought that my left leg was burned with blisters, I had to lie at home for nearly four months to cure the burns, but my left knee was left with lots of scars. This really could be described as 'I do not regret being pine away because of missing you'. This was my second realm.

After nearly two years of treatment, I became depressed, I lost the spirit to fight, no hope, only sadness, anxiety, and grievances. I almost lost hope on curing my legs and high blood pressure. At the end of August 2013, my wife found a program from somewhere for our daughter to lose weight. She told me solemnly that this program was not only quick and effective in losing weight immediately, but also worked well for blood pressure. I was full of doubt when listening to what she said. I thought that during the past two years, I had eaten whatever was claimed to be healthy, but blood pressure never went down. Yet, my daughter's dream of losing weight tempted me to try if I could lose my belly. So, with extreme suspicion, I began to implement Dr. Lu's program. Less than 20 days, my belly was gradually gone. When weighing myself, I found out that I lost about 10 kilograms, and my blood pressure also returned to normal range. What surprised me more was that my left leg pain, that had constantly brought me trouble and pain, was also gone.

This was called: 'after seeking for her for a thousand times in a thousand places, after looking back, she is standing under the dim lights.' In order to adjust the blood pressure and treat leg pain, I had gone through hardships, troubles everywhere, could not see any hope, but I did not expect the inadvertently carrying out this program would bring such a magical effect. So, I began to examine the program seriously, and I found that Dr. Lu's research results not only sorted out the real cause of obesity and Triple H, but also tried to cure the real cause of the problem, which undoubtedly brought hope to the Triple H and obese patients around China and around the world. Based on this, I have fully been involved in the promotion of this program and hoping to bring health, happiness and confidence to Triple H and obese friends around me, and also bring caring and happiness to the unfamiliar friends.

Comments:

Mr. Wu is a very resilient person, for the sake of health, it can be said he tried almost all of China's treatment means, including medicines, physical therapy, health care products. Although the results did not get worse, at least it did not get better. It is because these methods do not use human instincts adequately. Our direction is to seek inward, to find the answer in the life itself, so the direction of the whole program is to find people's instincts, and to restore people's innate function.

Case 8:

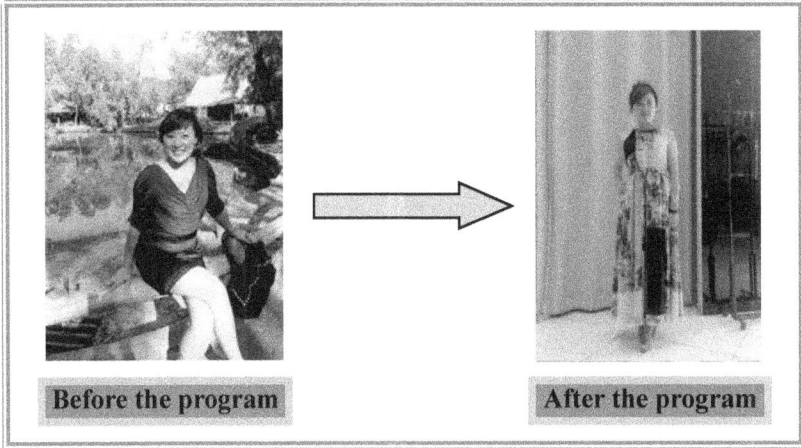

| Before the program | After the program |

My name is Jinying Li, born in 1978, height 167 cm, weight 65 kg, waist size about 90cm. I should have lived a carefree life every day at this age like my peers, but due to my physical problems, I felt fatigue both physically and mentally. With a history of 15 years of nervous headache, I had eaten pain tablets for more than 10 years. Due to genetic dietary reasons, I had gotten a bad heart disease which were more severe than the heart diseases sixty-year-olds get, mild fatty liver, gynaecological diseases etc.

On April 26 this year, I will never forget this day. I wanted to lose weight, and through the introduction of a friend, I started to implement Doctor Lu's program, wishing that I could have a wonderful summer this year. On the first day of the program, I had a severe headache, so I slept at 6.30pm till 6am the next day. My coach told me that I had a neurological headache, which was why it was more painful than normal headaches. This continued for three or four days, but then I started getting nausea as well. I could not even describe the feeling of vomiting, it was like being pregnant. No matter what I ate, I puked. Then my coach said, this was due to a poor liver, I knew that I had mild fatty liver, but in order to adjust the body I had to endure. And after three days, I thought I should be fine and the nausea and headaches should be gone. Yet, who knew there was a greater challenge ahead of me. My body itched so much that I could not even put the feelings in words. I woke up every midnight, I scratched myself so much but it did not work. When I could not stand the torture, I would wish that I could use a knife to peel off my skin, but I still carried on. I had been going through like this for 10 days. Now when I think of it, I still feel unpleasant. The coach said it was due to bad lungs, plus allergic skin, so it was more difficult for me to adjust than others. Yes, I was a skin allergy patient 10 years ago, when it was severe, I could only drink water, and there was nothing I could eat, but I did not think that it would appeared again during the treatment after so many years. After skin allergy, followed by lower back pain, I felt like I was cut in half. The coach said it was adjustment responses brought by gynaecological diseases. Tortured by diseases and pain one after another, I suffered a lot.

However, the adjustment results really made me surprised and happy, weight loss was the smallest return. I am now in a good mental state, I used to sleep for two hours at noon but I feel energetic without taking the nap; I used to have headache if I didn't have enough sleep but now the symptom is gone, most importantly, my heart disease is also cured. Before I walked very slowly, and it was hard to breathe if I walked a little faster. Now I can walk 130 steps per minute, and I can walk for an hour without panting, this is what excited my family. My fatty liver was gone, sometimes I drink with my friends on purpose, and I have found that I can drink a lot more than before. Gynaecological disease was also gone and I went to the hospital to have a comprehensive check, everything was normal. A healthy person cannot empathize with how happy a patient feels when the diseases are cured. Now, I weigh 57.5kg, and I have maintained it for 3 months. I also have become prettier, and more energetic. After experiencing the good results, I have started to recommend this program to my parents, siblings, and they all took part in this method and had good result. Every time I talk about it, I am very excited like because I feel like I now have magic.

It is this program that has brought me health.

It is this program that has brought me joy.

It is this program that has brought me happiness.

Case 9:

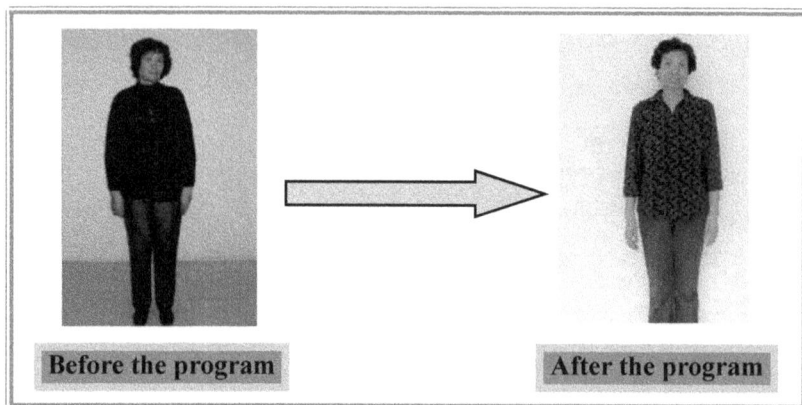

My name is Suhua Su, from Beijing. The followings are the data before and after I took part in Doctor Lu's program.

	Before program	After program
Weight	75.2kg	63.5kg
BMI	26	22.5
Waistline	83cm	80cm
Low-density lipoprotein	4.71mmol/L	3.83mmol/L
Total cholesterol	7.4mmol/L	6.15mmol/L
Creatinine	114.47μmol/L	104.31μmol/L
Uric acid	478.93μmol/L	404.85μmol/L
Glucose	6.2mmol/L	5.2mmol/L
PH	5.0	5.5
Epithelial cells (EC)	23.3/μL	7.3/μL
Epithelial cells (high power) (EC)	4.2/HPF	1.3/HPF
Fatty liver	Moderate	Mild

My adjustment experience was like this: I am 61 years old this year, an educated youth in Northeast Construction Corps in the late 1960s. I returned to Beijing due to nephritis caused by fever in the late 1960s. Due to the special time period (1960s) and special working environment, my body had accumulated a lot of problems when I was young. After I returned to Beijing and started a family. Because I had a lot of siblings and my parents I had to support, I overworked. I had high blood pressure, then obesity, hyperlipidaemia, hyperuricemia, moderate fatty liver, gastritis, lack of blood supply to heart and brain, and moderate cerebral infarction, when I was in my forties.

On April 17, 2013, because of an enthusiastic invitation from friends, I decided to try Doctor Lu's program, and travelled for one hour to arrive there. The program lasted for one and a half das, it was an incredibly happy journey. It was truly amazing! I ate six meals a day, but I lost 1kg without feeling hungry! After repeatedly consulting the coach, I decided to stick to it! A miracle happened! On the fourth day, I stopped my pill for high blood pressure and the blood pressure is 130mmol/L in the morning and 70mmol/L at night. On the 20th day, I increased the dosage to one pill a day due to a slight fluctuation, and stopped on the next day till this day (September 23). I did not take any more pills. During the program, I had the side effects of diarrhoea, cramps, bowel, and pain against my temples, insomnia and so on. Yet as time went by, the symptoms disappeared, all indicators approached to the normal range, and I lost 11.7 kg. I feel relaxed and energetic. It was Dr. Lu's program which allowed me to rejuvenate the youth!

I want to express my thanks to the coach for the warm and patient help and meticulous and thoughtful service. Thanks to this effective health management plan which greatly improved my body! Now, I dedicated to it and I feel happy when I do it. Meanwhile I hope that more and more people can join Dr. Lu's plans to improve their quality of life, improve health and wisdom, so that each of us really achieve health and happiness.

Before the program

民航总医院

姓名: 苏素花　　门诊手册: 10031498　　申请医师: 张晓苏　　科别: 中医专家
性别: 女　　标本种类: 血清　　检验科: 生化免疫室　　申请日期: 2012-11-27
年龄: 60 岁　　床　号:　　初步诊断:

No 项目	结果	单位	参考值		No 项目	结果	单位	参考值	
1 *钾(K)	4.42	mmol/L	3.5~5.5		21 *谷丙转氨酶(ALT)	17.95	IU/L	5~40	
2 *钠(Na)	142.19	mmol/L	135~150		22 *谷草转氨酶(AST)	20.01	IU/L	5~40	
3 *氯(Cl)	106.40	mmol/L	94~110		23 *碱性磷酸酶(ALP)	75.92	U/L	42~105	
4 二氧化碳总量(TCO2)	25.81	mmol/L	22~32		24 *γ-谷氨酰转肽酶(GGT)	14.40	U/L	10~40	
5 *钙(Ca)	2.32	mmol/L	2.03~2.54		25 *肌酸激酶(CK)	115.62	IU/L	25~170	
6 *磷(P)	1.23	mmol/L	0.96~1.62		26 肌酸激酶同工酶MB(CKMB)	13.38	IU/L	0~25	
7 镁(Mg)	0.97	mmol/L	0.8~1.2		27 *乳酸脱氢酶(LDH)	196.47	IU/L	114~240	
8 *葡萄糖(GLU)	6.20	mmol/L	3.9~6.1	↑	28 α-羟丁酸脱氢酶(HBDH)	138.73	IU/L	76~195	
9 *尿素氮(BUN)	4.62	mmol/L	2.2~7.2		29 HDL/CHOL	0.20		0.23~0.47	↓
10 *肌酐(Cr)	114.47	μmol/L	44~97	↑	30 间接胆红素(IBil)	16.61	μmol/L	0~18	
11 *尿酸(Ua)	478.93	μmol/L	149~387	↑	31 白蛋白/球蛋白比例(A/G)	1.55		1.0~2.5	
12 前白蛋白(PA)	241.30	mg/L	160.0~360.0		32 尿素氮/肌酐	0.06		0.03~0.10	
13 总蛋白(TP)	75.84	g/L	60~80		33 阴离子间隙	12.89	mmol/L	7.0~16.0	
14 白蛋白(ALB)	46.11	g/L	35~55		34 球蛋白(GLB)	29.73	g/L	20~30	
15 *总胆固醇(Chol)	7.40	mmol/L	3.6~6.0	↑	35 AST:ALT	1.11		0.8~3.0	
16 *甘油三酯(TG)	1.76	mmol/L	0.33~1.8						
17 高密度脂蛋白(HDL)	1.49	mmol/L	1.20~2.39						
18 低密度脂蛋白(LDL)	4.71	mmol/L	2.1~3.12	↑					
19 总胆红素(TBIL)	20.21	μmol/L	2~19	↑					
20 直接胆红素(DBIL)	3.6	μmol/L	0~6.84						

采样时间: 2012-11-27 10:23　　标本接收时间: 2012-11-27 10:46　　报告时间: 2012-11-27 14:19
备 注:　　操作者: 杨静　　审核者:
此检验结果只对该检验标本负责!

After the program

2013-06-06　　生化常规(一)

北京市医疗机构临床检验结果报告单　　No: 232

民航总医院

姓名: 苏素花　　门诊手册: 10031498　　申请医师: 张晓苏　　科别: 中医专家
性别: 女　　标本种类: 血清　　检验科: 生化免疫室　　申请日期: 2013-06-06
年龄: 60 岁　　床　号:　　初步诊断:

No 项目	结果	单位	参考值		No 项目	结果	单位	参考值	
1 *钾(K)	4.30	mmol/L	3.5~5.5		20 直接胆红素(DBIL)	4.3	μmol/L	0~6.84	
2 *钠(Na)	147.30	mmol/L	135~150		21 *谷丙转氨酶(ALT)	17.85	IU/L	5~40	
3 *氯(Cl)	110.20	mmol/L	94~110	↑	22 *谷草转氨酶(AST)	21.49	IU/L	5~40	
4 二氧化碳总量(TCO2)	28.87	mmol/L	22~32		23 *碱性磷酸酶(ALP)	59.22	U/L	42~106	
5 *钙(Ca)	2.44	mmol/L	2.03~2.54		24 *γ-谷氨酰转肽酶(GGT)	9.59	U/L	10~40	↓
6 *磷(P)	1.26	mmol/L	0.96~1.62		25 *肌酸激酶(CK)	111.33	IU/L	25~170	
7 镁(Mg)	0.99	mmol/L	0.8~1.2		26 肌酸激酶同工酶MB(CKMB)	10.96	IU/L	0~25	
8 *葡萄糖(GLU)	5.20	mmol/L	3.9~6.1		27 *乳酸脱氢酶(LDH)	200.95	IU/L	114~240	
9 *尿素氮(BUN)	7.24	mmol/L	2.2~7.2	↑	28 α-羟丁酸脱氢酶(HBDH)	146.03	IU/L	76~195	
10 *肌酐(Cr)	104.31	μmol/L	44~97	↑	29 HDL/CHOL	0.22		0.23~0.47	↓
11 *尿酸(Ua)	404.85	μmol/L	149~387	↑	30 间接胆红素(IBil)	16.05	μmol/L	0~18	
12 前白蛋白(PA)	218.43	mg/L	160.0~360.0		31 白蛋白/球蛋白比例(A/G)	1.62		1.0~2.5	
13 总蛋白(TP)	73.80	g/L	60~80		32 尿素氮/肌酐	0.07		0.03~0.10	
14 白蛋白(ALB)	45.65	g/L	35~55		33 阴离子间隙	8.23	mmol/L	7.0~16.0	
15 *总胆固醇(Chol)	6.15	mmol/L	2.80~5.18	↑	34 球蛋白(GLB)	28.15	g/L	20~30	
16 *甘油三酯(TG)	1.91	mmol/L	0.56~1.7	↑	35 AST:ALT	1.20		0.8~3.0	
17 高密度脂蛋白(HDL)	1.37	mmol/L	1.04~1.55						
18 低密度脂蛋白(LDL)	3.83	mmol/L	2.1~3.37	↑					
*高危人群 <2.59; 极高危人群 <2.07									
19 总胆红素(TBIL)	20.35	μmol/L	2~19	↑					

采样时间: 2013-06-06 08:58　　标本接收时间: 2013-06-06 09:20　　报告时间: 2013-06-06 13:15
备 注:　　操作者: 姚建民　　审核者: 姚建民
*高危人群: 冠心病、缺血性卒中/一过性脑缺血发作、糖尿病、慢性肾病、高血压合并三项危险因素　极高危人群: 急性冠脉综合征或任意两项高危因素合并存在。

Comments:

At the beginning of the program, various signs of improvement can occur to some people, but then gradually disappear, this is a very common situation. Signs of improvements mean that the hidden diseases or hidden danger have been removed from the body. Like the drain is blocked for many years, it is often very smelly when it is clearing, but after that it becomes clean and smooth.

The struggle between the vital energy and the pathogenic factor inside the body sometimes are at an equilibrium. The pathogenic factor does not completely crush you down, and vital energy does not complete get rid of pathogenic factor to restore the health. The body is in a state of feeling awful every day but still manage to bear it, until your body is completely crushed at last. Side effects are to take the initiative during the stalemate stage to support vital energy, to improve immunity, and to break the balance, finally to get rid of the disease. The sooner the process of experiencing side effects, the better it is. When your physical fitness still allows you, launch a campaign in time to completely restore your health. If you postpone it until you get old and weak, you will be strong in will but weak in power, you can only finish the final journey of life with diseases throughout your body

Case 10:

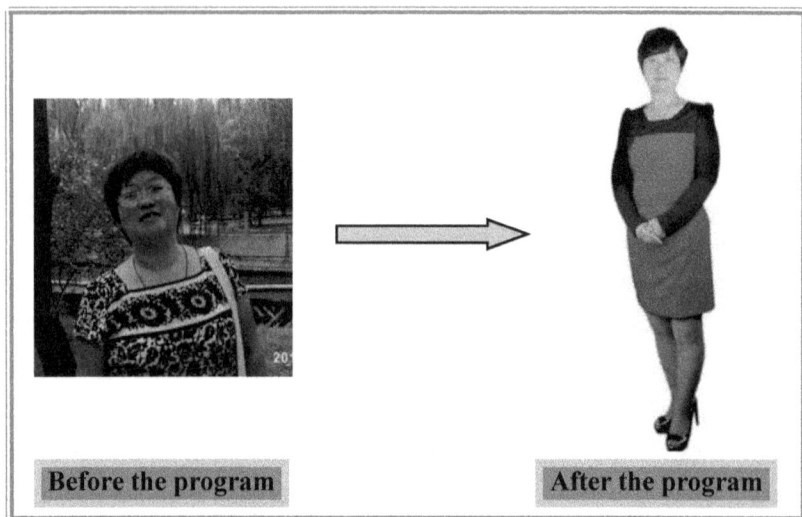

Before the program → After the program

My name is Zhaomei Li, born in 1968 in Jinzhong, Shanxi. Because I had to manage my business for many years, I ate irregularly, stayed up all night, and overworked, and all these resulted in serious endocrine disorders. For past two or three years, I had dysfunctional uterine bleeding. It made my menstrual periods to last for more than ten days each, which resulted in haemorrhagic anaemia. When it was at its most serious, I only had 3.5 grams of haemoglobin, and had to resort to blood transfusion. Strengthlessness, lower extremity swelling and dark facial spots visited me. I tried many Traditional Chinese Medicine prescriptions, and tried a lot of healthcare products, although the situation was slightly relieved, there was no fundamental change.

I began Dr. Lu's program on September 4, 2012. At the end of September my menstrual period lasted for 5 days (it was normal for the first time after the program), the second month lasted for 6 days, and the third month was for 5 days. It is completely normal now. My weight decreased from 82.5 kg to 69 kg in the first cycle and to 60 kg in the second cycle. I have lost 22.5 kg for two short cycles, which really makes me happy and excited. I have new hope for life and full confidence in life.

I have decided to join this industry, and make more people like me to regain the confidence and strength for life again. My greatest wish is to make women in the world healthy, beautiful and confident, to make more family happy and harmonious, and to make more people move towards healthy.

Comments:

Menstruation is a like a barometer of women's health. All kinds of factors that harm health will bring menstrual disorders, such as fatigue, cold, angry, shock and so on. The program turns waste into energy. Because it turns fat into the raw materials for cell reduction, tissue regeneration, organ recovery and body improvement. After weight loss, chi (a.k.a. energy) and blood, liver and kidney, hormones etc. are all adjusted comprehensively, and the menstrual is improved as a result.

Case 11:

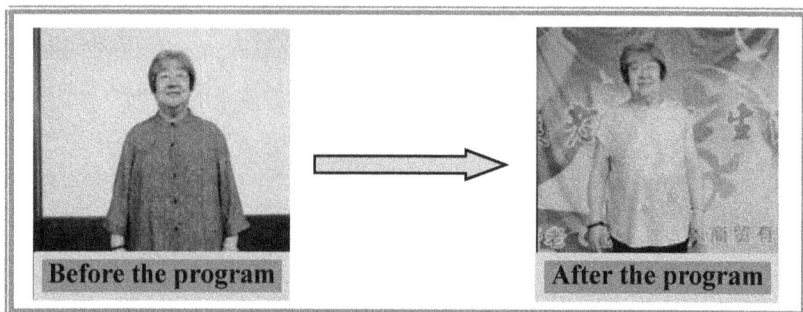

My name is Lianhui Zhang, from Beijing. Below is the data of my body before and after I participated in Dr. Lu's program:

	Before program	After program
Weight	82kg	68kg
Waistline	100cm	90cm
Blood pressure	150/90	130-140/80
Total cholesterol	5.70	4.52
Triglycerides	2.43	0.96
Fatty liver	Moderate	Mild

My name is Lianhui Zhang, 66 years old, 82 kilograms, I suffered from a variety of diseases: heart insufficiency, systemic arteriosclerosis, hypertension, high blood lipids, impaired glucose tolerance abnormal, moderate fatty liver, multiple lacunar cerebral infarction, Alba degeneration, gallbladder calculus and coronary heart disease. In 1989 my left kidney was removed due to kidney tuberculosis. So, my legs had oedema year in year out, I had to urinate three to four times a night, chronic gastritis, colitis and so on. Over the years I had been living in pain, which made my life very depressing.

What was more, I felt tired all day long due to difficulties in moving caused by physical obesity. I have tried a variety of ways to lose weight but all ended up with failures. The more I tried, the fatter I got. In particular, the experience of going to hospital to see a doctor was painful. I woke up at 3 o'clock to 5 o'clock in the morning for hospital registration, but the hope of finding a good doctor always never came true. Lots of pills didn't solve the problem, I looked at the pills in my hand, all sorts of feelings welled up in my mind. I actually ate the pills like food, but after that I didn't get any better and I had more diseases, and they were even more severe. Antihypertensive drugs increased from one tablet to four tablets per day. Being like this for a long time, liver function indicators became abnormal. But what else could I do? I had tried whatever I could try, but the effects were not good. I was really helpless, and just had to trust luck.

While I was in bitter pain, one day I heard about Dr. Lu's program. I wanted to try it out, so I participated in the experience camp in April 2013. A miracle happened within only one day, I lost 1.3 kg. In total, I lost 7 kg in 40 days. Blood pressure became stable, and I stopped taking antihypertensive drugs, fatty liver almost disappeared, I had normal blood lipids and normal blood sugar, leg swelling disappeared, chronic gastritis, and colitis also greatly improved. Changes in the body increased my confidence and I felt that health was waving to me. With confidence, I participated in the second cycle of short-term adjustment. Weight reduced by 14 kg to 68 kilograms. Due to the lack of blood supply of my heart before the program, I often felt chest pain, chest tightness, extrasystole, they were also greatly improved after the program. The colours of my lips turned from dark black to red. I feel relaxed when walking or doing work now. I have a good spirit now, as if I was a new person, the whole family was very pleased and supported me to continue the program. I am very grateful of this program as it gives us a way to find health. This is not only a means to health, but also the means to happiness.

Before the program

中国中医科学院广安门医院检验报告单

Guang An Men Hospital Affiliated China Academy of Chinese Medical Sciences

After the program

中国中医科学院广安门医院检验报告单

Guang An Men Hospital Affiliated China Academy of Chinese Medical Sciences

Comments:

It is a common phenomenon that cardiac function can be improved while improving obesity and Triple H. Although we still lack systematic data to prove the extent of improvement in cardiovascular dilation and myocardial blood supply, the patient's changes are already the best proofs. It is hypothesized that improvements in cardiac function stems are from three reasons:

The program promotes the body's own vascular dredging function;

Weight loss itself reduces heart load;

Chi and blood improvement indirectly improves blood supply to heart.

Case 12:

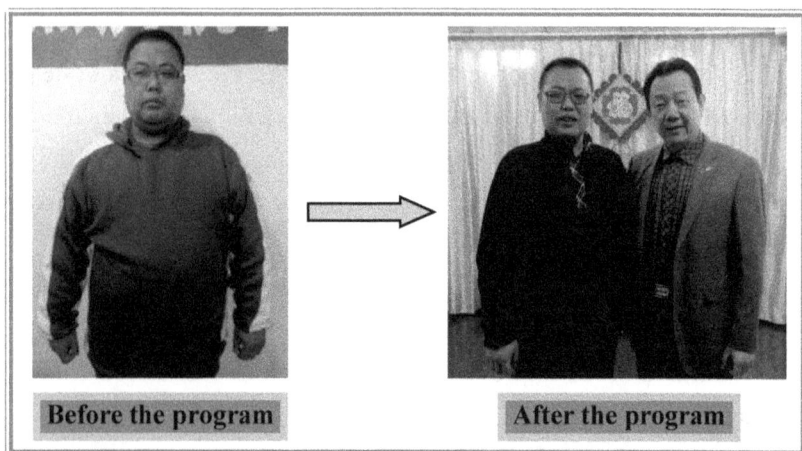

| Before the program | After the program |

My name is Xu Yang, 41 years old. I participated in health management because of a recommendation of my second eldest aunt Lianyu Zhang (disease category case 23). Because Lianyu Zhang and her six other sisters, including my mother, all had hereditary diabetes, my eldest aunt died of diabetes at an early age, and our family was living under a cloud because of this disease.

Fortunately, my second eldest aunt focused on health, over the years she had not given up, and asked for cures all around. By chance, she participated in the Dr. Lu's program, the effects were very good, insulin injections reduced from the original 103 units to now 19 units daily, and blood sugar, blood pressure, blood lipids, and blood uric acid all reached the standards. My aunt was in great joy and advised my mother and me to join in together. Was it as magical as she said? I began the program with doubt. What I didn't expect was that miracle happened the next morning. My original weight was 131.2kg and blood sugar is 8. In one day, I lost by 1.3kg and fasting blood sugar dropped to 5.8. The change was absolutely shocking.

Before this I actually felt my physical conditions were very bad. I was a chef, a few years ago, an accident injured my cervical and I had to give up my job. The physical pain and heavy life pressure led to my long-term insomnia. Later, the addiction to online gaming made tired all day long, I didn't want to do anything, and I didn't even want to shave my beard. I was in my poorest sate. Every day I went to the office, I just slept on the sofa, and often slept on the bus to the terminal bus station after finishing work. Sometimes my legs were swollen, I had knee pain and heel bone hyperplasia. At the company's physical examination, I was found that fasting blood glucose reached up to 8.0, I had severe fatty liver, and weighed 131kg.

The report was never opened and lied on my desk for six months, and it was my health coach who came to visit me and opened it. Why didn't I want to open my medical tests and look at the result? The reason was simple, I was afraid to open it, like how a lot of people do not dare to participate in a health examination. Our thoughts are very contradictory, I was young, and my child was only 8 years old. Health was very important to me, and if I collapsed at this time, my family would collapse with me. My mother had Triple H, and I wanted to take care of my parents. I had a child to raise and parents to take good care of, so it was an awkward age. I deceived myself on purpose, trying to fool myself that I was not sick. After participating in Dr. Lu program, I obtained good effects, my life rekindled with hope. I am a man who is not good at expressing my feelings, and in my mother's eye my health is more important than her own health, so I am going to say to my mother here, 'Mom, thank you for everything you have done for me.'

Today is the 240th days since I took part in the program, my weight reduced from 131.2kg to 92kg, successfully lost 39.2kg, almost 40kg. Fasting blood sugar was 5.3, fatty liver also disappeared. The most important effect is that I have become a man full of energetic and responsibility from a man without fighting will and even didn't want to speak. More importantly, I have no more addicted to virtual networks. It was Dr. Lu's program that saved me; the effects from the program were unexpected but it was the start of my rebirth.

I have not only got healthier, the most important thing is that I have learned the advanced healthy lifestyle. I will benefit from learning this health management for the rest of my life, and I will pass this kind of health ideas to family and friends. Thanks to this program, I would like to thank those who have helped me. This is a course that accumulates goodness, behaves goodness, benefits the country and the people, and creates a harmonious society. I will actively share this healthy way with more people, spread happiness, and meet more kind people, so that more people can improve the quality of their lives.

Comments:

Health is a responsibility, and you do not belong to yourself. If you give up, who will help you smooth your parents' endless sadness? If you collapse, who will replace you to love your partner and children? Out of responsibilities, we have to face the challenges, out of responsibilities, we have to be persistent and committed. Sometimes, the way to health is started with only a chance and a decision.

Case 13:

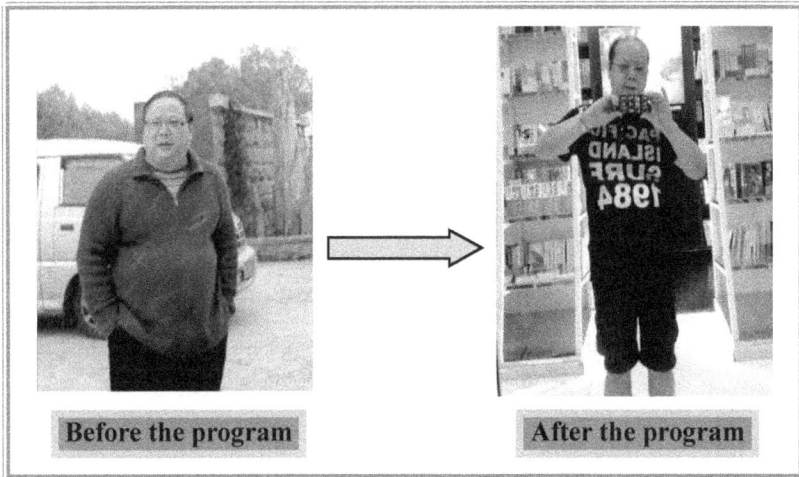

Before the program | After the program

I was a patient of metabolic syndrome for a long time, also overweight (the average weight from 1997 to 2013 was more than 95kg). Also, in June 2004, due to coronary artery occlusion which (had caused old myocardial infarction), I undertook an intervention therapy. For the therapy, a total of 7 stents were put into my body, which costed RMB 360,000 yuan (approx. $87,270 USD). During this period (1997 – 2013), I tried a variety of weight loss methods, such as exercise, diet, protein powder, medication, vegetable juice, slimming tea, bitter gourd and many weight loss products, with no effect and my weight reached record highs. Diabetes, high blood pressure, high uric acid, high blood lipids, coronary heart disease came one after another. Since then, I took various medicines for a long time, but the indicators were still difficult to control, and sometimes I thought these diseases and the fats would be with me for my whole life.

I implemented Dr. Lu program in June 2013, which showed effects quickly. I have developed a new way of life while losing weight. It has been nearly half a year with no rebound. Here's a review of the process of implementing Dr. Lu's program:

I boycotted this method at the start, as I had been in the medical industry for many years, and I did not believe that patients of diabetes and/or high blood pressure could get off drugs completely. I had tried countless weight loss methods, it was either that the effects were not obvious or it was easy to regain the weight, and if you didn't take special care, a little carelessness could increase the weight to a higher level than the original weight. So, I was sceptical about the weight loss effects of the program. With my friend's persuasion and encouragement, I decided to try, and adopted this program. The effects were clearly visible since the beginning. In the first two weeks, I lost 0.5kg per day (a total of 7kg). In the third week, a total reduction of 1kg. The slower decrease was because that I had hit a plateau, also, I did not do the exercises due to gout. I lost 3kg in the fourth week, a total of 10kg (from week 1 to week four). Through this experience, I really understood and established a new scientific concept, reconfigured a new lifestyle, I had more passion and confidence for life. In addition, after getting rid of 10kg (after more than ten years), my physical and mental pressure was eased, sleep had improved (I changed the bad habit of staying up late), energetic, and quit cigarettes (psychologically as well). Moreover, I stopped the pills for reducing blood pressure, blood sugar and blood lipids, without feeling any discomfort. My blood pressure became more stable. Sixty days after the program, I took a physical examination, the indicators were better than the indicators before the implementation of the program. Such as: severe fatty liver was gone, fasting blood glucose, which was more than 10 during medicine taking period, was 6.4 without medication after the program, almost within the normal range. Through personally experiencing the program, I am confident that Dr. Lu's approach to the establishment of a scientific lifestyle and regaining cell activity is correct, I believe in his method of reversing metabolic diseases. I believe that there will be more experiments to prove that metabolic diseases can get rid of drug dependence. May Dr. Lu's program bring healthy new lives to more people!

Comments:

The stent is an operation for coronary artery occlusion. The opening of the blocked or narrow blood vessels doesn't mean that coronary heart disease, myocardial infarction are cured. Strictly speaking, stent surgery is not a treatment, but a first aid measure. Carrying out a stent surgery is for more treatment time, the idea of which everything will be ok after putting in the stent is wrong. After the stent surgery, it is important to control the blood pressure, blood sugar, blood lipids, blood viscosity etc., if these four indicators cannot be maintained at a satisfactory level; the patient will face the risk of recurrence within half a year. The purposes of the program for Yong Li were: first, to reduce weight and reduce cardiac pressure load; second, to lower blood pressure, blood sugar, blood lipids, blood viscosity, and reduce the risk of recurrence.

Case 14:

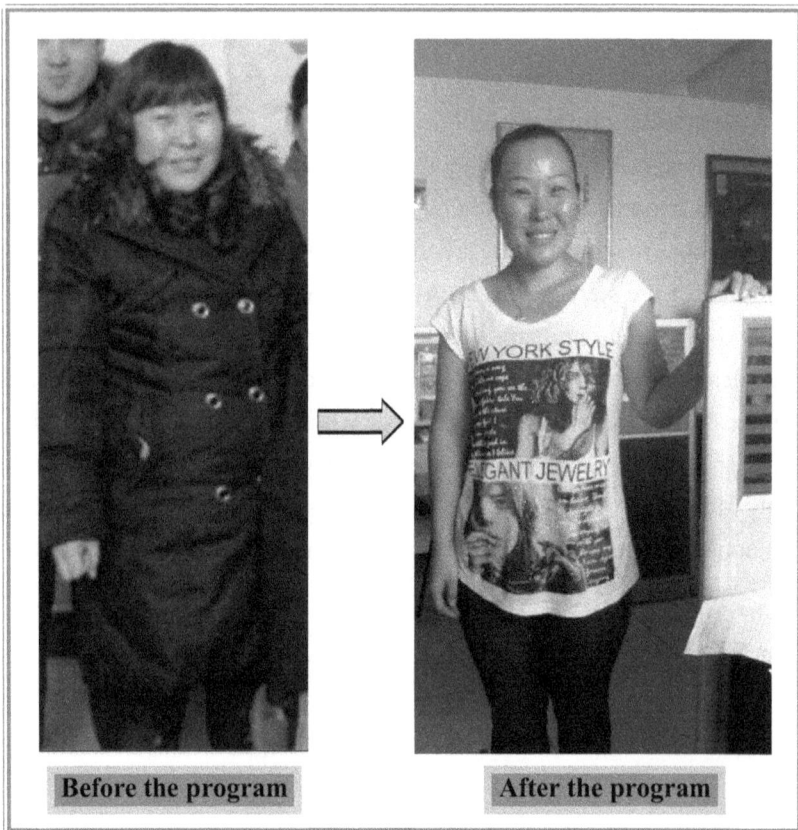

Before the program

After the program

Medical report before program

河北省直体检中心检验报告单

体检编号：20130.150019　姓名：魏彦丽　性别：女　年龄：32　单位：个人体检

检验人：卜军娟　　　检验日期：2013-03-15

生位	项目代号	项目名称	结果	单位	正常值范围	标志
	AST	谷草转氨酶	28	U/L	5.00	40.00	
	ALT	谷丙转氨酶	62	U/L	5.00	40.00	
	TB	总胆红素	9.5	umol/L	5.10	35.0	
	DB	直接胆红素	2.81	umol/L	0	6.80	
	TP	总蛋白	69.0	g/L	60.00	82.00	
	ALB	白蛋白	42.2	g/L	32	51	
	CHO	总胆固醇	5.45	mmol/L	2.84	5.18	
	TG	甘油三酯	6.17	mmol/L	0.4	1.70	
	HDL-C	高密度脂蛋白-Ch	1.03	mmol/L	1.04	2.0	
	LDL-C	低密度脂蛋白-Ch	2.17	mmol/L	1.90	3.37	
	BUN	尿素氮	3.13	mmol/L	1.700	7.10	
	CREA	肌酐	47.8	umol/L	44.00	123.0	
	UA	尿酸	286	umol/L	140.0	428.0	
	GLU	血糖	5.39	mmol/L	3.9	6.0	

Medical report after completing the first cycle

河北省直体检中心检验报告单

体检编号：201307010149　姓名：魏彦丽　性别：女　年龄：31　单位：个人体检

检验人：于明娟　　　检验日期：2013-07-01

生位	项目代号	项目名称	结果	单位	正常值范围	标志
	AST	谷草转氨酶	30	U/L	5.00	40.00	
	ALT	谷丙转氨酶	40	U/L	5.00	40.00	
	TB	总胆红素	11.7	umol/L	5.1	35.0	
	DB	直接胆红素	4.74	umol/L	0.00	6.80	
	TP	总蛋白	69.1	g/L	60.00	82.00	
	ALB	白蛋白	48.2	g/L	32	51	
	CHO	总胆固醇	3.33	mmol/L	2.84	5.17	
	TG	甘油三酯	1.24	mmol/L	0.40	1.70	
	HDL-C	高密度脂蛋白-Ch	0.66	mmol/L	1.04	2.00	↓
	LDL-C	低密度脂蛋白-Ch	2.17	mmol/L	1.90	3.37	
	BUN	尿素氮	5.25	mmol/L	1.70	7.10	
	CREA	肌酐	58.7	umol/L	44.00	123.0	
	UA	尿酸	246	umol/L	140.00	428.00	
	GLU	血糖	4.45	mmol/L	3.90	6.00	

石家庄市第四医院

黑白 超声医学影像报告单

JL-YI-213

超声号：

| 姓名：魏彦丽 | 性别：女 | 年龄：31 岁 | 初复诊： | 科别：门诊 |
| 病历号： | 住院号： | 病区号： | 床位号： | 费用： |

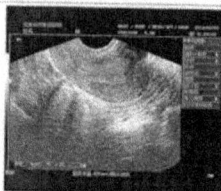

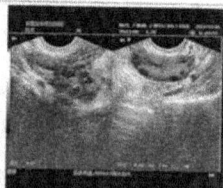

超声所见：
1. 膀胱充盈情况 TVS
2. 子宫图像
   子宫位置 后 位 大 小 4.7*4.5*3.2 厘米
   内膜厚径 0.47 厘米
   宫壁回声均匀
3. 卵巢影像
   右卵巢大小 3.9*2.5 厘米,可见约20个卵泡,较大0.7*0.6厘米
   左卵巢大小 3.3*1.7 厘米,可见约22个卵泡,较大0.5*0.5厘米
4. 其它情况
   子宫直肠窝 可见液性暗区厚约0.9厘米

诊断意见：
子宫正常大

本次超声检查报告仅代表本次检查结果,仅供临床参考,不属诊断依据,如特殊情况者,建议咨询临床医师并动态观察随诊。

徐州市宝河医疗设备有限公司

记录：王雪青   诊断医师：李娜

检查时间：2013-07-05 11:05

只作临床参考,不作证明材料

Medical report after completing the second cycle

河北省直体检中心检验报告单

| 体检编号：201308270086 | 姓名：魏彦丽 | 性别：女 | 年龄：31 | 单位：个人体检 |

检验人：于明娟   检验日期：2013-08-27

生化	项目代号	项目名称	结 果	单位	正常值范围		标志
	AST	谷草转氨酶	22	U/L	5.00	40.00	
	ALT	谷丙转氨酶	25	U/L	5.00	40.00	
	TB	总胆红素	17.7	umol/L	5.1	35.0	
	DB	直接胆红素	6.03	umol/L	0.00	6.80	
	TP	总蛋白	69.4	g/L	60.00	82.00	
	ALB	白蛋白	47.4	g/L	32	51	
	CHO	总胆固醇	3.48	mmol/L	2.84	5.17	
	TG	甘油三脂	0.93	mmol/L	0.40	1.70	
	HDL-C	高密度脂蛋白-Ch	1.08	mmol/L	1.04	2.00	
	LDL-C	低密度脂蛋白-Ch	2.21	mmol/L	1.90	3.37	

My name is Yanli Wei, 31 years old, I am a cosmetics company brand assistant. Two years ago, due to overwork, stress, long-term travelling, irregular lifestyle and diet, my physical conditions were worsened. I had severe night sweats, insomnia, a lot of dreams, menstrual disorders, rheumatoid arthritis, back pain (could not stand the pain after bending over one minute), arm numbness and other symptoms. After a period of therapy with Traditional Chinese Medicine, the problem didn't improve much, but I became fatter. My weight went from 59kg to 81.5kg. Later, I had even more problems: snoring, breast hyperplasia and other symptoms.

In April 2013, I learned from a friend that Dr. Lu's program has helped a lot of Triple H and obesity patients, and my friend suggested me to a physical examination, saying that it would be useful for comparison in the future. I was interested, so I went to do the physical examination. The results thunderstruck me. I had severe fatty liver, excessive transaminase, hyperlipidaemia, high cholesterol and other symptoms. I tried to start the first cycle, and lost 1.2kg the very first day. The next day I didn't sweat during sleep, and the quality of sleep became good. On the third day, my husband said that I wasn't snoring. On the sixth day, my period came, the colour of the blood was much better, the amount also increased. I lost a total of 3.3kg in the first week. I continued on with the program. Signs of improvement in joint pain, sleepiness and bloating and other reactions slowly appeared, then gradually disappeared. My second period came after 32 days, there was a lot more than the first time, the stomach was not so cold. For the first cycle of short-term plan, I lost 13kg. I went to physical examination again, only high-density protein was still a bit low, high cholesterol and high cholesterol had disappeared, severe fatty liver became mild, my complexion was much better than before, back pain disappeared. I was really happy, I thought the program was amazing. I could not wait to carry out the second cycle of the program. During the second cycle, joint pain, sleepiness, palpitation chest tightness and other symptoms were all gone, the body became lighter and lighter, a variety of symptoms slowly disappeared, the third and fourth period came as scheduled, with a normal colour, and lasted for 4 days compared with one day before the program. I went to have a physical examination at the end of the second cycle, and the result were very good and all the indicators were normal, fatty liver also disappeared. Gynaecological examination indicates that the polycystic ovarian follicle also reduced, breast hyperplasia completely disappeared. Weight reduced from 81.5kg to 55.5 kg. In April 2014, a great surprise came - I was pregnant! The doctor said that people suffering from polycystic ovarian follicles would become infertile, and it was a miracle that I could get pregnant. I would like to thank God for letting such beautiful thing happened to me!

I'm really grateful for the program, it let me to start a beautiful and healthy life. I hope that more friends who have had the same experience (before the program) can open up their hearts, and implement this program, they should get to know more about it, and then benefit from it.

Comments:

Ms. Wei's gynaecological problems have improved significantly with the metabolic changes. Gynaecological problems are a part of the reflections of the overall problem, which is to say that because the overall health is not good, the gynaecological problems cannot be cured. When the overall health is improved, gynaecological problems would also improve. This also confirms how scientific Doctor Lu's program is.

Case 15:

Hello everyone! My name is Yuan Zhang, 36 years old, from Tianjin, I am in the financial industry.

At end of 2012, the pressure from work, family and other aspects, caused my body to be unhealthy. All kinds of diseases came one after another. I didn't know what to do, I was so physically weak at such a young age, so I often felt melancholy. With the introduction from my friend about the training program of Dr. Lu, my parents and I started the program at the same time. After the adjustment, we had a physical examination each. The day of getting the medical report was important to me because that day was my birthday (March 7th, 2013). When I saw the medical results, I cried. The abnormal indicators which used to show on my parents' reports went normal. This was really a great birthday gift!

My 65-year-old father (Shaowu Zhang) had gotten cerebral infarction 10 years ago. In the past 10 years, he received infusion regularly every spring and autumn. Yet, the fingertips numbness still had not been improved, and he walked slowly, and the friction between his shoes and the ground could often be heard. After program, he walks much better than before, there is no more sounds of the friction between shoes and floor, and his face has turned brighter, also with a good mental state.

It is worth mentioning that, because of my family's improvements, there have been five friends joining the plan. We have not just done a physical therapy, but also have started the journey of understanding ourselves, caring for ourselves, and finding for health.

	Before program	After program
Weight	85.6kg	76.1kg
Triglycerides	2.26	1.16
Uric acid	420.5	368.7
Blood pressure	150/106	128/80
High-density lipoprotein	0.73	0.85

Father's medical report before program

Father's medical report after program

Comments:

Ms. Zhang's father had gotten cerebral infarction 10 years ago, thus inconvenience in walking. They were improved after the program. Also stroke sequela alleviated. This case shows that the brain cells after stroke can be properly restored. The old medical theory held that brain cells could not be regenerated after the cells die. Yet, the latest medical experience has shown that these brain cells are not dead but dormant. That is, if some kind of means can re-activate the sleeping cells, some of the brain function can be restored. This program aims at taking care of human instincts, to restore human instinct. This case proves that this program is not only useful to the regeneration of the various organs in the body, but also activate the brain cells regenerate.

Case 16:

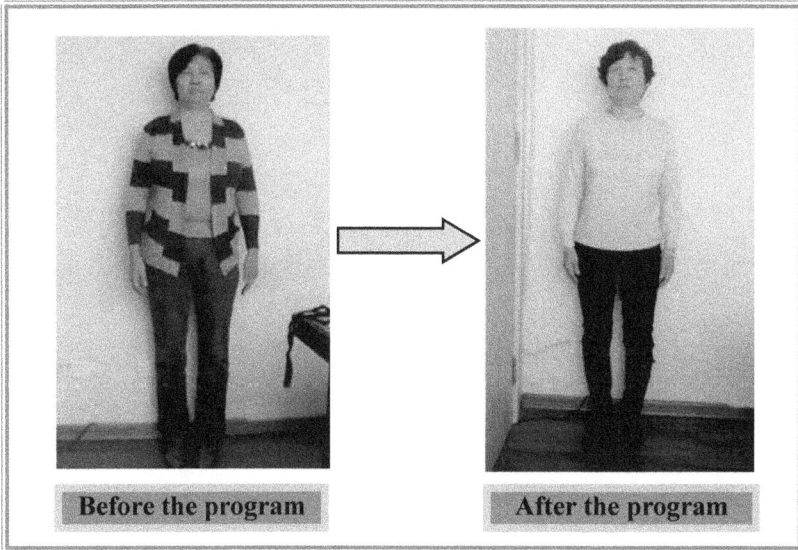

Before the program → After the program

My mother is 61 years old (written by Yuan Zhang) (Wang Wenying, Zhang Yuan's mother), but the once cheerful mom became chit-chatty, forgetful, stubborn, bad tempered after menopause. I suspected that she had mild depression, but we could not find any suitable solutions after researching. After Dr. Lu's program, my mother started smiling again, her attitude became optimistic and cheerful again, and as considerate as before. All these surprised me.

	Before program	After program
Weight	68.2kg	61,1kg
Triglycerides	100cm	90cm
Low-density lipoprotein	4.04	3.07
Glutamic oxalacetic transaminase	48.5	26.7
Glutamic-pyruvic transaminase	48.9	32.4
R-glutamyl transpeptidase	57.5	29.2

Mother's medical report before adjustment

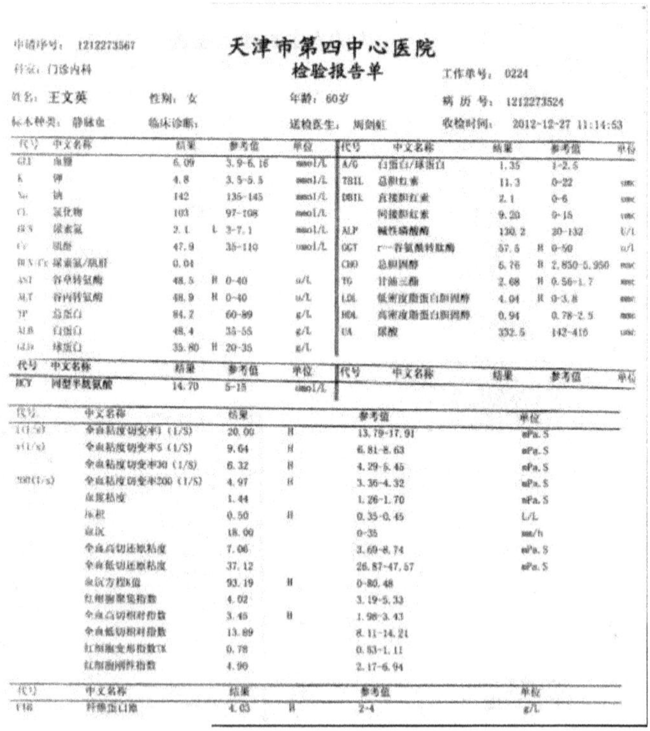

天津市第四中心医院
检验报告单

申请序号：1212273567
科室：门诊内科　　工作单号：0224
姓名：王文英　　性别：女　　年龄：60岁　　病 历 号：1212273524
标本种类：静脉血　　临床诊断：　　送检医生：[illegible]　　收检时间：2012-12-27 11:14:53

代号	中文名称	结果		参考值	单位
GLU	血糖	6.09		3.9-6.16	mmol/L
K	钾	4.8		3.5-5.5	mmol/L
Na	钠	142		135-145	mmol/L
CL	氯化物	103		97-108	mmol/L
BUN	尿素氮	2.1	L	3-7.1	mmol/L
Cr	肌酐	47.9		35-110	umol/L
BUN/Cr	尿素氮/肌酐	0.04			
AST	谷草转氨酶	48.5	H	0-40	u/L
ALT	谷丙转氨酶	48.9	H	0-40	u/L
TP	总蛋白	84.2		60-89	g/L
ALB	白蛋白	48.4		35-55	g/L
GLB	球蛋白	35.80	H	20-35	g/L

代号	中文名称	结果		参考值	单位
A/G	白蛋白/球蛋白	1.35		1-2.5	
TBIL	总胆红素	11.3		0-22	umc
DBIL	直接胆红素	2.1		0-6	umc
	间接胆红素	9.20		0-15	umc
ALP	碱性磷酸酶	130.2		20-132	U/L
GGT	r-谷氨酰转肽酶	57.5	H	0-50	u/l
CHO	总胆固醇	6.76	H	2.850-5.950	mmc
TG	甘油三酯	2.68	H	0.56-1.7	mmc
LDL	低密度脂蛋白胆固醇	4.04	H	0-3.8	mmc
HDL	高密度脂蛋白胆固醇	0.94		0.78-2.5	mmc
UA	尿酸	332.5		142-416	umc

代号	中文名称	结果	参考值	单位
HCY	同型半胱氨酸	14.70	5-15	umol/L

代号	中文名称	结果		参考值	单位
1(1/s)	全血粘度切变率1 (1/S)	20.00	H	13.79-17.91	mPa.S
5(1/s)	全血粘度切变率5 (1/S)	9.64	H	6.81-8.63	mPa.S
	全血粘度切变率30 (1/S)	6.32	H	4.29-5.45	mPa.S
200(1/s)	全血粘度切变率200 (1/S)	4.97	H	3.36-4.32	mPa.S
	血浆粘度	1.44		1.26-1.70	mPa.S
	压积	0.50	H	0.35-0.45	L/L
	血沉	18.00		0-35	mm/h
	全血高切还原粘度	7.06		3.69-8.74	mPa.S
	全血低切还原粘度	37.12		26.87-47.57	mPa.S
	血沉方程K值	93.19	H	0-80.48	
	红细胞聚集指数	4.02		3.19-5.33	
	全血高切相对指数	3.45	H	1.98-3.43	
	全血低切相对指数	13.89		8.11-14.21	
	红细胞变形指数TK	0.78		0.53-1.11	
	红细胞刚性指数	4.90		2.17-6.94	

代号	中文名称	结果		参考值	单位
FIB	纤维蛋白原	4.03	H	2-4	g/L

Mother's medical report after adjustment

Comments:

Ms. Zhang's mother changed from bad tempered before the program to smiling every day after the program, which shows that people are physically and mentally integrated. Physiological conditions determine the psychological condition. Physical health will bring mental health, and thus health intervention on the body brings personality changes.

Case 17:

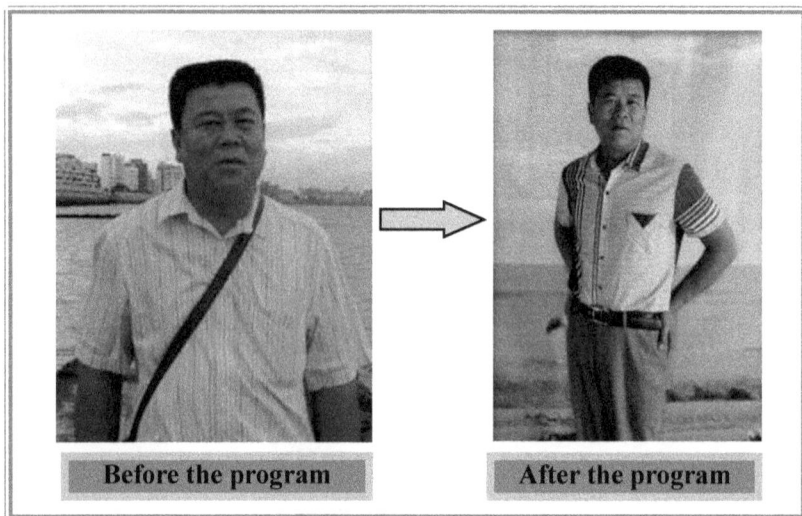

Before the program → After the program

Good things are determined by destiny, and my destiny with this program began on a train. It was July 2011. I met a coach on the train, after a conversation, I learned that this program could make people to lose 5kg to 15kg in one month, and helped Triple H patients get rid of 70% -80% of drug dependence after one cycle of adjustment. I thought that since it had such good effects in such a short time, I shall have a try too.

At that time, my waist size was 1m, weight was 85 kg, blood lipids, blood pressure, uric acid, transaminase, transpeptidase were above the normal standard. When eat I could not swallow down the food, I could not maintain my life through such a basic way, which really depressed me. I always felt that I had oesophageal cancer or some bad diseases like that, and felt that I could only live for three or five more years. Knowing this piece of information, I did not care whether the claimed effects were true or not, I had to try. I would rather bear the disappointment of failure than not trying at all. I was not willing to give up hope without even trying. I participated in training camp in September 2011.

In order to verify the effects of this program, throughout the program, I made four Comprehensive Metabolic Panels, signs of improvements were shown each time. After the program, all of my body indicators were within a normal range, with a weight loss of 15 kilos, blood lipids from 4.11 to 1.11, blood pressure before adjustment was 100/130 whereas after adjustment was 80/120, transaminases 99 to 29, transpeptidase 120 to 33, uric acid 550 to 330. I felt old previously, now I felt young and vigour. Before I felt that I only have three to five years to live; now I felt that I could live to 100 years old.

It has been three years after I finished the program, my weight has been maintained between 67.5 kg and 69 kg. So, I have brought this method back to Handan, so that my friends, relatives and folks in Handan can also have a healthy body. I am here to thank this program which can benefit mankind. I am grateful for coach's watchful guidance, and I hope that more friends not only benefit from it themselves, but also help their friends and relatives to benefit as well. In this way, we are also doing a favour for the mankind. Good people deserve good returns, and will go smoothly in their life. I wish everyone a healthy and happy life.

10 days after program

After one cycle

Comments:

Through the comparison of data of the above case, we can see that many indicators have a downward trend. However, it should be noted that this program is not to blindly lower the indicators. If the indicators were reduced blindly, low blood pressure and low blood sugar would occur. The program is to restore the normal functions of the human body.

The program does not reduce Triple H indexes, but rather, it restores the body's metabolic indicators to a normal range. In the course of the program, indicators which are below the safety range can also be improved, rather than simply reducing the number.

During the implementation of the program, the general principle of the using of hypoglycemic drugs and antihypertensive drugs is to reduce the amount gradually. There is a small part of the younger participants with short disease course who can stop drug within a day. Whereas older participant with long disease duration can only reduce the dosage but cannot stop fully. The rest of the people can gradually reduce the intake of drugs, and normally, within one week or one month, one can completely stop medicine. The principle of reducing the drug goes with the reduction of blood glucose and high pressure. If there is no decline in blood glucose and high pressure, dosage is not reduced; if there is a decline, then dosage is reduced. If the dosage is not decreased when the blood pressure and blood glucose have decreased, then there will be hypoglycemia or low blood pressure, similar to how normal people will have hypoglycemia, low blood pressure when taking medicine. The part that has been reduced corresponds to the restored function of the body part.

Case 18:

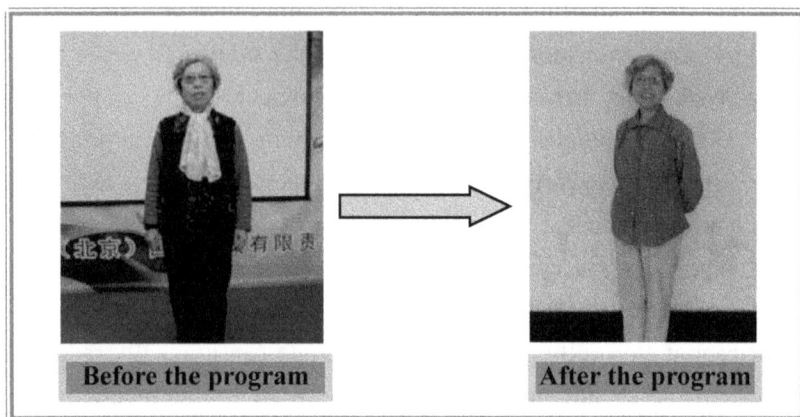

| | Before the program | After the program |

My name is Lianyi Cheng, from Beijing, below is the physical data before and after I participated in Dr. Lu's program:

	Before program	After program
Weight	50.9kg	49kg
Urine protein	+++	N/A
Urine occult blood	+++	N/A

Hello everyone! My name is Cheng Lianyi, a retired soldier, 70 years old. By chance, I got to know Dr. Lu's program. The first time when I listened to the coach's introduction of the program, I was very sceptical, and thought that the effects were impossible. At that time, my belief was that if you felt unwell, you shall go to the hospital, and conduct drug treatment. So, having a lot of trusts in the hospitals, I had visited many big hospitals in recent years. The doctors gave me a lot of Chinese and Western Medicine, and I took a handful of drugs every day. It had been three consecutive years like this, but the treatment effects were unsatisfactory. I sincerely hoped that the conditions of my body could improve. I often recalled when I was young, I was so valiant in the army, but now my body was deteriorating. My spirit was not good, I felt sad and emotional, along with my husband passing away, I felt very down.

I live with my son now, because my physical condition was very bad, my children were very worried. Then, I saw a lot of patients like me had a good body restoration through Dr. Lu's program. Some lost several kilos, some even stopped antihypertensive drugs, but didn't have to inject insulin. I was very surprised and curious! So, I tried the personalized plan, designed by my coach, of fruit and vegetable juice. After a cycle, when checking in the hospital, the urine protein, urinary occult blood became normal compared to the three pluses before, and I was very surprised when I received my examination report. I could not believe that it had such good effects. I thought that there might be errors in the data, after reconfirming with the doctor that the numbers were correct, and I was very happy and excited!

A month later, my daughter-in-law saw my body changes, and she was very curious, taking the initiative to consult me. I was also very pleased to introduce this program to her. After a short-term strengthening, she lost 7.5kg, and her mental state changed obviously. She used to feel very tired after coming back home from work, she did not want to move after coming home, she didn't feel like doing anything. In contrary, now she doesn't feel tired and with good spirit, she very active in doing the housework.

I am a soldier and I treat my life seriously, I only say what is true. The above is what really happened to me. I am more than 70 years old this year, I really appreciate this program from the core.

Before the program

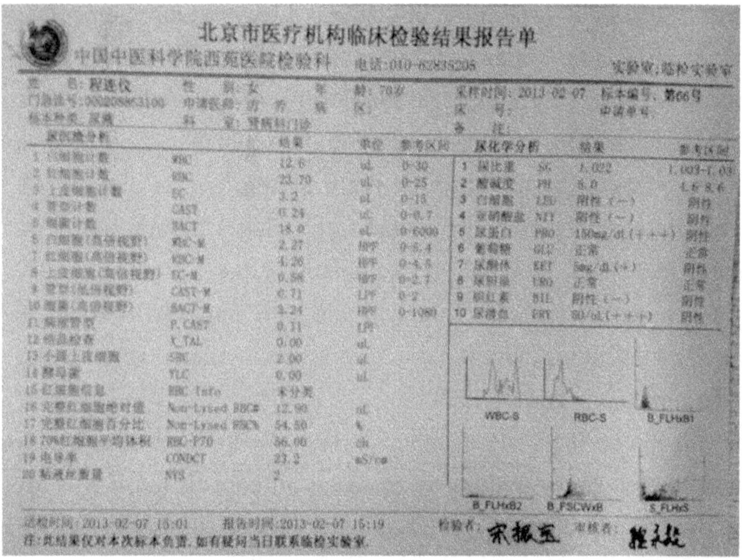

北京市医疗机构临床检验结果报告单

中国中医科学院西苑医院检验科 电话:010-62835205 实验室:临检实验室

姓名:程连仪 性别:女 年龄:70岁 采样时间:2013-02-07 标本编号:第66号

门急诊号:000208863100 申请医师: 病区: 床号: 申请单号:

标本种类:尿液 科室:肾病科门诊 备注:

尿沉渣分析		结果	单位	参考区间
1 白细胞计数	WBC	12.6	uL	0-30
2 红细胞计数	RBC	23.70	uL	0-25
3 上皮细胞计数	EC	3.2	uL	0-15
4 管型计数	CAST	0.24	uL	0-0.7
5 细菌计数	BACT	18.0	uL	0-6000
6 白细胞(高倍视野)	WBC-M	2.27	HPF	0-5.4
7 红细胞(高倍视野)	RBC-M	4.26	HPF	0-4.5
8 上皮细胞(高倍视野)	EC-M	0.58	HPF	0-2.7
9 管型(低倍视野)	CAST-M	0.71	LPF	0-2
10 细菌(高倍视野)	BACT-M	3.24	HPF	0-1080
11 病理管型	P.CAST	0.31	LPF	
12 结晶检查	X_TAL	0.00	uL	
13 小圆上皮细胞	SRC	2.00	uL	
14 酵母菌	YLC	0.00	uL	
15 红细胞信息	RBC Info	未分类		
16 完整红细胞绝对值	Non-Lysed RBC#	12.90	uL	
17 完整红细胞百分比	Non-Lysed RBC%	54.50	%	
18 70%红细胞平均体积	RBC-P70	56.00	ch	
19 电导率	CONDCT	23.2	mS/cm	
20 粘液丝数量	NYS	2		

尿化学分析		结果	参考区间
1 尿比重	SG	1.022	1.003-1.03
2 酸碱度	PH	6.0	4.6-8.6
3 白细胞	LEU	阴性(-)	阴性
4 亚硝酸盐	NIT	阴性(-)	阴性
5 尿蛋白	PRO	150mg/dl(+++)	阴性
6 葡萄糖	GLU	正常	正常
7 尿酮体	KET	5mg/dl(+)	阴性
8 尿胆原	URO	正常	正常
9 胆红素	BIL	阴性(-)	阴性
10 尿潜血	ERY	80/ul(+++)	阴性

送检时间:2013-02-07 15:01 报告时间:2013-02-07 15:19 检验者: 审核者:

注:此结果仅对本次标本负责,如有疑问当日联系临检实验室。

After the program

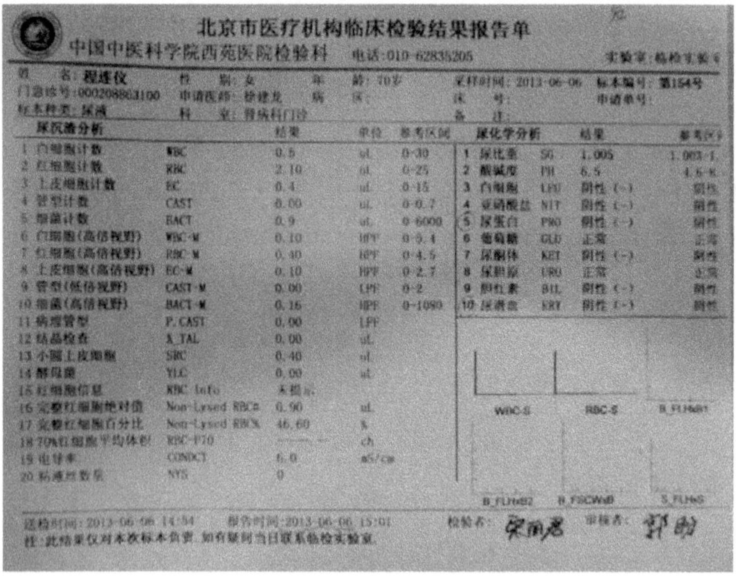

北京市医疗机构临床检验结果报告单

中国中医科学院西苑医院检验科 电话:010-62835205 实验室:临检实验室

姓名:程连仪 性别:女 年龄:70岁 采样时间:2013-06-06 标本编号:第154号

门急诊号:000208863100 申请医师: 病区: 床号: 申请单号:

标本种类:尿液 科室:肾病科门诊 备注:

尿沉渣分析		结果	单位	参考区间
1 白细胞计数	WBC	0.5	uL	0-30
2 红细胞计数	RBC	2.10	uL	0-25
3 上皮细胞计数	EC	0.4	uL	0-15
4 管型计数	CAST	0.00	uL	0-0.7
5 细菌计数	BACT	0.9	uL	0-6000
6 白细胞(高倍视野)	WBC-M	0.10	HPF	0-5.4
7 红细胞(高倍视野)	RBC-M	0.40	HPF	0-4.5
8 上皮细胞(高倍视野)	EC-M	0.10	HPF	0-2.7
9 管型(低倍视野)	CAST-M	0.00	LPF	0-2
10 细菌(高倍视野)	BACT-M	0.16	HPF	0-1080
11 病理管型	P.CAST	0.00	LPF	
12 结晶检查	X_TAL	0.00	uL	
13 小圆上皮细胞	SRC	0.40	uL	
14 酵母菌	YLC	0.00	uL	
15 红细胞信息	RBC Info	[illegible]		
16 完整红细胞绝对值	Non-Lysed RBC#	0.90	uL	
17 完整红细胞百分比	Non-Lysed RBC%	46.60	%	
18 70%红细胞平均体积	RBC-P70	——	ch	
19 电导率	CONDCT	6.0	mS/cm	
20 粘液丝数量	NYS	0		

尿化学分析		结果	参考区间
1 尿比重	SG	1.005	1.003-1.
2 酸碱度	PH	6.5	4.6-8
3 白细胞	LEU	阴性(-)	阴性
4 亚硝酸盐	NIT	阴性(-)	阴性
5 尿蛋白	PRO	阴性(-)	阴性
6 葡萄糖	GLU	正常	正常
7 尿酮体	KET	阴性(-)	阴性
8 尿胆原	URO	正常	正常
9 胆红素	BIL	阴性(-)	阴性
10 尿潜血	ERY	阴性(-)	阴性

送检时间:2013-06-06 14:54 报告时间:2013-06-06 15:01 检验者: 审核者:

注:此结果仅对本次标本负责,如有疑问当日联系临检实验室。

Comments:

Ms. Cheng used our supplementary program. The urine protein reflects the problems in the kidneys, and occult blood reflects the problems in the kidneys or bladder. The auxiliary program plays two roles:

1. Cleaning the blood and reducing the kidney pressure load. The kidney is the organ that filters the blood and produces urine. The dirtier the blood, the greater the burden on the kidneys. It is important to reduce load to restore the kidneys, just like how the most important thing is to not carry any heavy stuff when the shoulder is injured due to carrying heavy things. Only then we will have opportunity to cure.

2. Providing adequate raw materials to speed up tissue regeneration. Whether it is urine protein or occult blood, it is because something that should not be leaked is leaked. Glomerular need to be repaired, and the raw materials they need cannot fully come from medication, but also from food. Adequate nutrition supports the repair of damaged tissue, and as a result, the urine protein and occult blood would disappear.

Case 19:

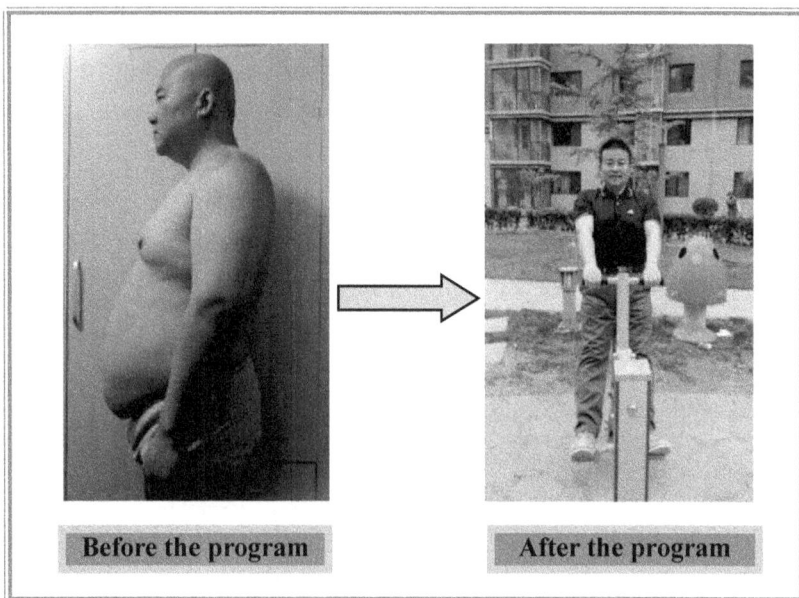

| Before the program | After the program |

'Huan Liu Junior' Enjoys Life because of Doctor Lu's Ten Years of Hard Work

Gang Lu is my real name. In my social circle, people refers to me as 'Huan Liu Junior' (p.s. Huan Liu is an overweight Chinese singer). I like to sing Huan Liu's song since childhood, and currently I work in China Broadcasting Art Troupe, I am a State Class-Two Artist. Doctor Lu and I have been friends for more than ten years. In 2002, we went to Hong Kong together to learn about nutrition and each got an advanced nutritionist qualification certificate.

Obesity had been torturing me, not just life inconvenience, but also took a lot of opportunities away from me. In fact, there had been a lot of important performances and my leader strongly recommended me to take part in them, but the director rejected me subtly after looking at my body shape, which weighed more than one hundred kilos. So, I missed my chances one after another. Alas, if was is not for obesity, I would have been Class-One artist. I felt very regretful that I had missed so many opportunities and the only consolation was the satisfaction from food. Due to long-term overeating, in 2008 and I got diabetes, since then, diabetes had been haunting me, and the complications of diabetes attacked me.

In 2014, I participated in the training camp held in Shunyi, Beijing. The side effects of the program were severe. During lectures, I was very sleepy. On the second day, I weighed myself and it turned out that I lost 1.8kg! I was astonished! After coming back home, I spent two days to go through Doctor Lu's data. On the third day after coming home, I invited the coach to my house, I said that I intended to devote the rest of my life to promote this program! This time, the coach was shocked! I made this decision not by impulse。 The decision is because that I am surprised to see how Dr. Lu has focused on this matter for ten years, and finally we have found a solution, and the method is very useful and brilliant. I trust Dr. Lu a lot! He has not only solved the problems that cannot be solved by overseas experts, but also has reached a higher level in the theoretical level, which I really admire!

I'll now share with you how I witnessed the miracle.

I stopped blood sugar drugs on the first day of the program, the blood sugar level reduced from 7.8 to 5.7 in one week. Now my blood sugar is stable at 4.6 ~ 5.0. My vision is no longer blurry. My left eye vision improved by 50 degrees (i.e. 20/200 to now 20/150). Vision is wider than before, the situation of shedding tears when facing the wind has disappeared, and floaters in the right eye has become much better than before. Hair has started growing out again, hair loss phenomenon has completely disappeared. Oil and messy hair has disappeared. My face has turned from dull to bright, as if I am ten years younger than before. Before I took my children to Happy Valley, a lot of people asked if my children were my grandchildren. Once, there was someone on the bus offered to give me a seat because he thought I was very old. A few days ago, I took my children to Taoranting (a place in China) to play the Big Slide, others said that I had become younger, and I played crazier than my son, that feeling was really good! I am a totally new me mentally and psychologically, I have become very confident after getting rid of diabetes that had been with me for 6 years, and I am now away from the threat of complications of diabetes. I am no longer the fat person that I was for 20 years.

Joint pain has disappeared, my body has become lighter. The pain that had troubled me for many years has completely disappeared after 25 days into the program. Then I have put away cupping machine, massage machine, field effect treatment instrument, that I used to use every day, from somewhere near the bed to a cupboard. Once my son and I took the subway home. When we arrived the southwest entrance of Nan Li Shi Road, there was no elevators. I got my son to have a race with me up the stairs. My ten-year-old son did not take this as a race, because had never won such kind of games, but the results shocked both my son and me. There were three landings from top to bottom of the staircases. When I rushed to the last tread, my son had only reached the first landing. I heard a phrase that I hadn't been heard for a long time: 'Father, waiting for me!' My eyes welled up.

I used to eat too much, I had a big appetite, and I could eat a KFC Family Sized Bucket by myself. I must go to sleep after dinner, as I always felt too tired and too sleepy. After program, my appetite is much smaller than before, nor greedy, and more energetic than before. When I first started dancing, I felt like I could not catch up with the rhythm, but now I feel the pace is too slow, I can add one extra move for every four beats.

Due to greatly enhanced immunity, I once saw a buddy downstairs, I only wore a short-sleeved top and thin pants out! When I came back, I ran into my neighbours from downstairs. She said 'You have a good body, it is zero degree outside, are you not cold?' I laughed with pride and said that I was used to this, if it was before, I would caught a cold. After 10 days of the program, I experienced morning wood that had been absent for a long time which greatly improved the quality of my sex life.

My weight before the program was 107.8kg, and it was reduced by 16 kg after one 42-day cycle. The skin is not loose. Yet, my belly, arm and legs have some marks, like a woman's stretch marks. Before program my belly looked like as if there were many of red earthworms lying there, and now they have turned lighter, thinner, and some have become one thin line, which is the evidence of the old fat me. The doctor said that a lot of fat people who had lost weight would have those marks, they would never disappear. I thought it was not big deal; just let them be the evidence of my past.

Many people asked me that after I had lost by 15kg really quickly, wouldn't it affect my singing? Would I be able to catch my breath? When I get asked such questions, I sing the final highest note for 20 beats from the song 'My Sun' as a response. After listening to my singing, they all clapped hands without questioning. Yet, once I sang the sad song 'Homesickness' with a cheerful sweet tone. My students said that my emotion expressions were wrong. I said that I could not feel sorrow anymore, I was happy every day now. How wonderful is the world, how wonderful is life!

My ideal weight is 65kg. I will implement two more cycles of the program to reach my goal. My heart is full of gratitude and thanks: I know for sure that Dr. Lu had suffered a lot during the one-decade long development of this program, but he was never willing to give up because of focus and dedication. Fortunately, the work has paid off, and he has overcame all of the obstacles, and gave everyone a solution to solve the problem. I, as one of the many beneficiaries, want to express my wholehearted gratefulness! The achievements of Dr. Lu have a transcendental significance. I am willing to take it as my lifelong career.

Comments:

It is a common phenomenon to reduce appetite after the program. Some people mistakenly think that the stomach becomes smaller, but the fact is that energy orbit is restored. Before the program, due to incorrect tracks, the nutrition cannot be successfully delivered to the cells. Although one may eat normally, but the cells do not get nutrition. The nature of hunger is cell hunger. For example, if we eat meat every day, we will yearn for vegetables, because the cells lack of vitamins and minerals. If we eat boiled cabbage every day, we will long for meat, because the cells lack of protein and fat.

Because the cells are hungry, although the stomach is full, but we still need to eat, it is like as if there was an endless hole in the stomach. In particular, we yearn for staple food (technically, it is because cells require the high glycaemic index food to stimulate insulin secretion to deliver more blood sugar to the cells), which is called 'carbohydrate addiction.' After the program, due to orbital recovery, when we eat normally, the nutrients can be successfully delivered to the cells. Because the needs of the cells have now been met, the appetite is naturally reduced, and energy is improved.

This carbohydrate addiction usually takes 1-2 weeks to be treated. Yet some people will stop the plan because they crave for staple food. Therefore, rational awareness oneself and encouragement from are conducive for success of this stage. After that, building a new lifestyle will become easier and easier.

After the program, morning wood is a normal phenomenon. Causes for impotence, such as diabetes, fatty liver, obesity and other factors, are eliminated. At the same time, the body becomes healthy, and full of energy, the morning wood comes naturally.

Case 20:

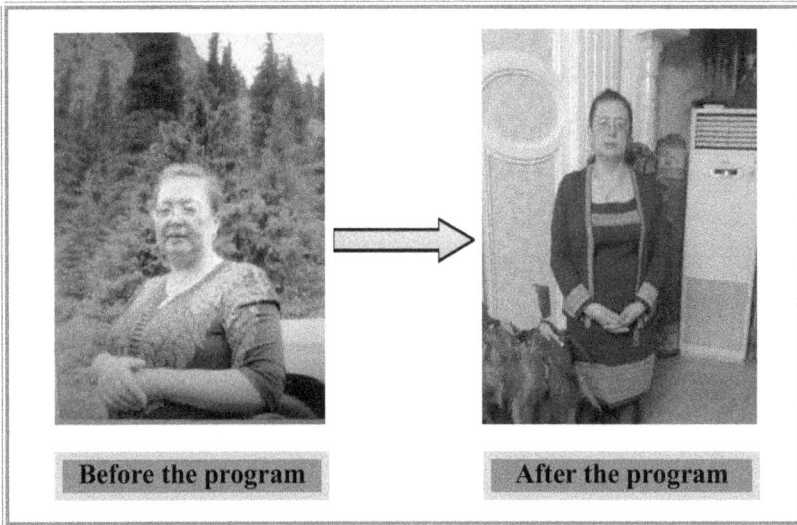

| Before the program | After the program |

I am 'Adalaitiabudoukadi', 50 years old, comes from Xinjiang Urumchi Uygur. I had been suffering from depression, and hospitalized at the end of 2013. When I left, the doctors gave me prescriptions for one-year dosage: everyday, a pill of 'Zelite', 'Roller' half pill, a quarter of 'Si Ruikang'. Thus, drugs were important in my life.

Waking up every morning to see these large and small bottles, it became the start of my bad mood of the day. Sometimes I thought that I could not never get rid of these drugs in the future, but luckily, I met Dr. Lu's plan. This is a plan difficult to describe by language, but it has improved my serious insomnia, cured my depression. After starting the plan, I strictly followed the plan for a month, and it really had significant effects. I stopped all the medicine, and lost 11kg. Loose skin became tight, spots were gone, and my skin even became paler and softer. Many of my friends looked at me with suspicion and thought I had a plastic surgery in Korea. It boosted my confidence to become even healthier.

What was unexpected was that menstrual period stopped for two years after an operation. After the program, menstrual periods came back again. Thanks to Dr. Lu's plan, it saved me. It gave me health, beauty and confidence!

Comments:

The major feature of this program is that everyone who is experiencing the program will have really good moods, depression can be improved significantly. We are not very clear of the mechanism, but it is certain that the changes of the body play a very big role to the changes in the mentality.

Case 21:

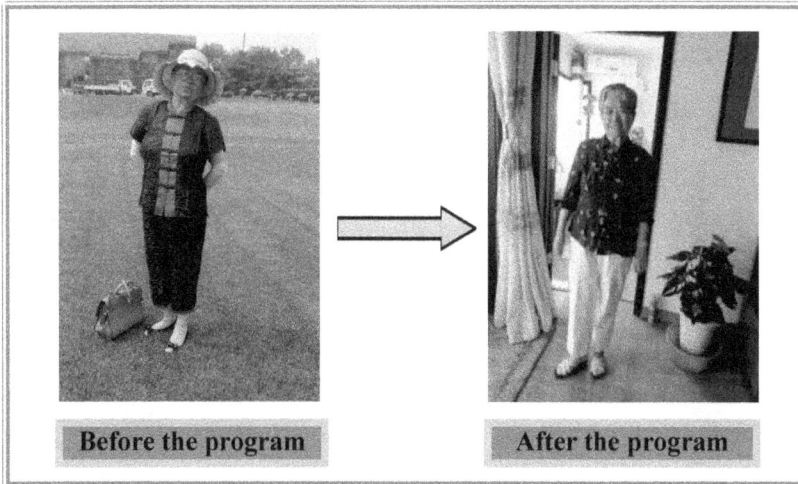

| Before the program | After the program |

My name is Yulan Zhao, from Beijing. The changes in my physical data before and after the program are as below:

	Before program	After program
Weight	61.1kg	56kg
Hip size	3	2.8
Waist size	2.45	2.27
Blood pressure	160/90	123/69

My name is Yulan Zhao, now 72 years old, I live in Zhujiang Junjing Residential Community of Muxiyuan. I have superior living conditions, the children are very nice, my husband also treats me well, and all these make me feel like that I am a happy woman. Yet, before the program, the fly in the ointment was that I suffered from high blood pressure, from the one pill to three pills. Although I knew that eating these pills could greatly hurt my kidney, I dared not stop them, and it had been four years. My blood pressure was still unstable. Sometimes was 160/90, sometimes was 140/90 and it made me felt stressed and worried.

By chance, I got to know a new health management method when participating in activities, and I heard that it could improve Quadruple H (hypertension, hyperlipidaemia, hyperglycaemia, hyperuricemia), assist cell reduction, and restore human instinct. I was overjoyed, and listened to the coach patiently when he gave me a detailed introduction, and told that I had the opportunity to experience. My husband was very understanding, and said that there was not need to just experience, as long as it worked, we would join, and he immediately decided to join with me.

In next few days, except from the basic tests, we also did a Comprehensive Metabolic Panel according to requirement. On July 7, my husband and I started the first day of the program. It was awkward on the very first day. The eating habits for years were suddenly changed, although we were not hungry after meals, it felt weird. Our coach communicated with us every day about the situation, because we had not taken the lectures, we had a poor understanding towards the new diet change. In the next day, my husband began to eat snacks secretly, because I was responsible for reporting to the coach every day, I told the coach this. Then the coach gave us a one-and-a-half-day training camp. My husband and I learned very carefully, and understood why our old eating habits were wrong, and knew why we had to eat like how the program told us to. After going home, my husband packed all the snacks and sent them to our coach, and we still strictly enforced the program every day. Soon after 42-days-short-term program was over, I lost 4.9kg, but the effects of body shaping were good. Others said that I looked younger. Notably, my blood pressure medicine was stopped 30 days into the program, and this was what I would not dare to think of before. I was very pleased. At the end of September, I took my granddaughter, who came back from Canada for her summer vacation to join the adjustment. My granddaughter was seriously overweight. At the moment, the effects seem pretty good. I am grateful to the R & D (research and development) staff of this project, for letting my family and me to benefit from this program. At the same time, I hope that more patients can benefit also, because the 21st century we compete not for money, but for health.

Meanwhile, I sincerely hope that friends all over the country are happy and long-lived!

Comments:

Ms. Zhao is a typical middle-part obesity, not overweight, but her waist size surpassed the danger line (greater than 80cm), and there are a lot of people like this. The program is concerned more on obese in middle part of the body but not obesity overall. Middle-part obesity is the most important manifestation of insulin resistance. When the energy paths are corrected, and insulin resistance reverses, the waist size certainly drops below the danger line. In addition, middle-part obesity also means that there is too much visceral fat in internal organs; reduced waist size means that visceral fat is removed.

Case 22:

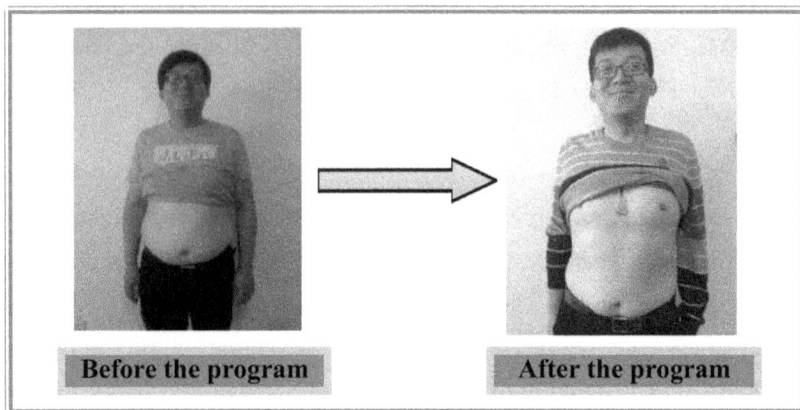

| Before the program | After the program |

My name is Guangpeng Ruan，29 years old. I'm a young man who has just become a father. I was fat since I was a child and suffered from familial genetic hypertension, and the highest blood pressure could reach up to 150/100, so I needed to take antihypertensive drugs every day; I also suffered from severe fatty liver, I felt tired all day, and I became very lazy and didn't feel like exercising at all. Because my condition was not good, I usually behaved tired and bored towards everything, so gradually, there were some conflicts in the family. I had a strong sense of health care since taking up the health industry in 2010, then I had tried nursing my body, but the effects were not good.

I was lucky enough to attend the training camp in 2013 June when I was extremely worried. Before that, my weight was 113kg, the blood pressure was 150/100, and I suffered from severe fatty liver. The next morning, my weight dropped 1kg and my blood pressure also returned to normal, which boosted my confidence. And then I had continued and finished the entire short-term program. Now my weight is 90kg and I have lost 23kg successfully. The blood pressure has been kept at around 120/80. A few days ago, I was informed by the hospital's health check that my severe fatty liver has become mild. I look like another person.

I cannot wear my old clothes because they are so big and the clothes I wear now are all newly bought. Wearing my dream clothes size makes me feel very contented. The most gratifying thing is that my mental state has recovered a lot, and I am not sleepy every day now. Unlike before, I was sleepy all day and fell asleep as long as there was a place to sit. In comparison, I don't feel sleepy from the time I wake up in the morning until I got to bed at night, and I become better at my work. I love sports now, and my family is very happy for me. I didn't feel any pain in the entire adjustment cycle, and there is no sign of rebound after 200 days.

Comments:

Almost all obese people know that they should exercise more, but most of them cannot do it. Why are all of them so 'lazy'? Because the method is wrong, the tissue cells cannot get nutritious, naturally they will not have vitality. This often manifests as lethargy, fatigue and poor health. The first step of this scheme is not to make people move, but to make cells alive. Once the cells restore their vitality, people, as a result, will have the energy to do exercise.

Chronic diseases are formed at the age of 25-45, so health interventions are the most critical at this stage. Mr. Ruan is the representative of Chinese powerful labour force, many of them lack energy and their efficiency is not high, which results in only partial utilization of their wisdom and ability. Although they are very aggressive, but incapable of action, and some even die at young age. Effective metabolic adjustment and the establishment of healthy lifestyle bring them not only the energy when they are young, work easiness, easy accomplishments in their careers, but when they are older, all of them can enjoy a good, peaceful life.

Case 23:

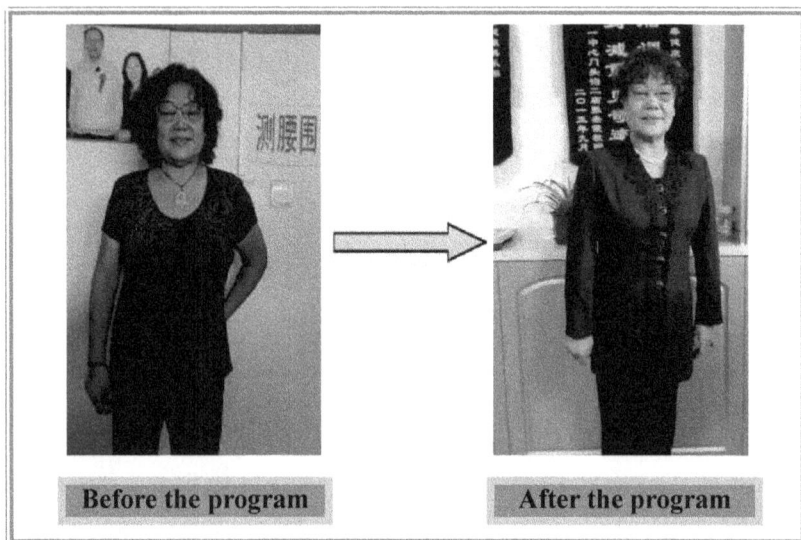

Before the program | After the program

My name is Lianyu Zhang, from Beijing, These are my physical data changes before and after taking part in the program of Dr. Lu:

	Before program	After program
Weight	75.8kg	69.1kg
BMI	28.5	26
Waist size	91cm	85cm
PBPI	150/70 mmHg	130/65 mmHg
GIs	14.6mmol/L	5.2mmol/L
Uric acid	438umol/L	396umol/L
Fatty liver	Moderate	Mild
Medication	77umol/L, 6 pills of hypoglycaemic drugs, 2 pills of hypotensive drugs	19umol/L, both hypoglycaemic and hypotensive drugs withdrew

I am 71 years old, from Beijing. I was suffering from hypertension, diabetes, high uric acid and fatty liver. I had had diabetes for 30 years; sometimes, up to 103 units of insulin were injected in one day. Before the program, I injected 77 units every day, took hypoglycaemic drugs and even went to the hospital for treatment and body check-ups many times, but the blood glucose could not be controlled and the fasting glucose level was 14.6mmol/L. Union Hospital doctors told me that there was no other way because I had developed insulin resistance, I had to have injections and take hypoglycaemic drugs. I lost all of my hopes.

On August 17th, I held a sceptical attitude and attended the health management training camp and finished 60 days of the program. My blood glucose has changed significantly. Currently, I have stopped taking the medicine and I only need to inject 19 units of insulin every day, and the blood glucose is controlled at around 5.2mmol/L. I am very happy and I would like to thank Dr. Lu's program for letting me to reclaim myself and life. I will certainly let my family and friends join this program quickly!!

Comments:

Most of diabetics have given up dreaming about recovery when they meet us because of the doctor's advice, and the doctor's view has a decisive effect on the patient.

This program is so effective, why doesn't the hospital use this? In fact, many domestic hospitals are aware of the important way of life, and even have set up a special department for nutrition, such as the Nutrition Department of Union Hospital was set up as early as 1921, when the hospital was established. Yet this area is still not considered as important. Moreover, in recent years, the explosive impacts of Lifestyle Disease have left the unprepared doctors and patients shocked. For example, diabetes was rarely found in China decades ago, and it entered a period of rapid growth after 2000, so it was a new disease. People are beginning to pay attention to diabetes and finding solutions in recent decades. Now the medical industry has realized that lifestyle has a major impact on diabetes and has begun to study simpler and more effective coping strategies. This book shows only first-stage research results, but we believe that the use of lifestyle to solve Lifestyle Disease will become a broad consensus, and simple and effective program will certainly be widely used.

Case 24:

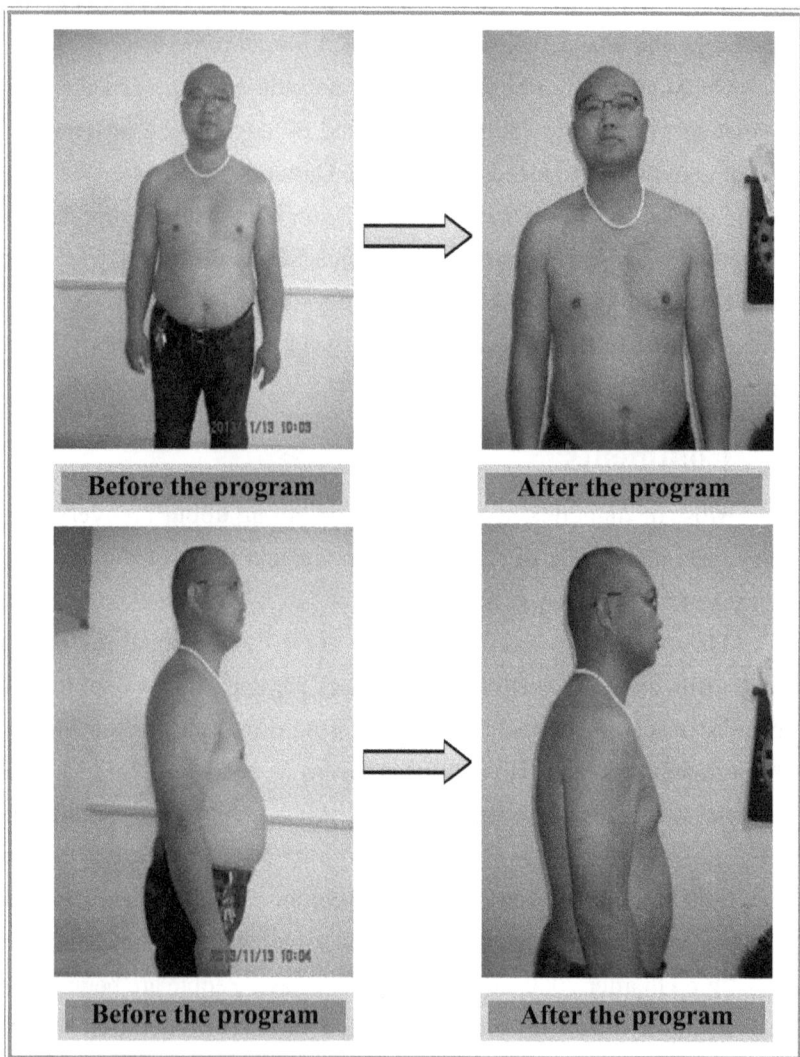

Before the program

After the program

Before the program

After the program

My name is Yong Li, I'm a 36 years old who has engaged in the health industry for 2 years, so I pay more attention to health. Despite that, I found that I was on the wrong track when I got to know Dr. Lu's program. It overthrows many of my previous perceptions. Although I was also nursing myself before, but my Comprehensive Metabolic Panel data really shocked me. Because there were a lot of data which had exceeded the standard, but I did not feel uncomfortable. I started the program on November 13th, 2013, and ended the short-term program after 42 days on December 25th, 2013. The statistics of my body were improved by this cycle of nursing, such as: before the program, 6 out of 11 of the indexes of liver functions were abnormal; after the program, only 3 out of 11 slightly exceed the standard; uric acid decreased from 614 to 425; triglycerides decreased from 3.88 to 1.04; Moderate fatty liver was also cured; weight changed from 110kg to 98kg with a successful loss of 12kg. This success has filled me with confidence so that I have not given up yet and am still keep going. I'm sure I'll be better and better.

Through more than a month of experience, not only did I gain a healthy body, but also realized that lifestyle changes had magical effects. This program is the best metabolic adjustment method I have ever seen because it has many advantages that general adjustment methods don't have. I would like to thank the R & D team, please allow me to say, 'thank you!' sincerely. Changing me makes my entire family. Making me healthy makes the entire family healthy. I would like to spread this good news to everyone around me, so that they will be healthy quickly!

Before the program

包头市第八医院

超声检查报告单

仪器型号：PHILIPS 检查日期：2013-11-15

姓名：李勇 性别：男 年龄：38 岁 超声号：206 住院号： 病区床号：

科别：内1 申请医生：王志文 临床诊断：待查

检查部位：肝胆脾胰

告知：超声检查受诸多因素影响，如自身因素（肥胖、气体干扰、准备欠佳、配合差）、病变位置特殊、疾病所处不同阶段等）、设备因素（仪器型号及性能不同，其图像质量量有差异）、检查者因素（超声结论依据国内外公认的影响特征，对图像的判读不同检查者之间可能存在差异）等。此报告是影像检查结果，请以病理诊断或临床最后诊断为准，与检查相关的医疗活动应您予了解上述结果并与临床医生沟通。

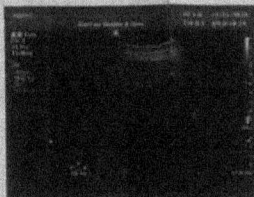

超声摘述：

肝脏大小、形态未见异常，包膜完整，肝缘光滑，内部声前方增强，后方衰减，肝内血管走行正常，门静脉内径正常。

胆囊大小正常，形态规则，囊壁光滑，内透声好，肝总管无扩张。

脾大小形态未见异常，包膜完整光滑，内回声均匀，脾静脉内径正常。

胰腺形态大小未见异常，包膜完整，内部回声均匀，主胰管无扩张。

超声诊断： 脂肪肝

Test report after 20 day's adjustment

Adjustment after 32 days

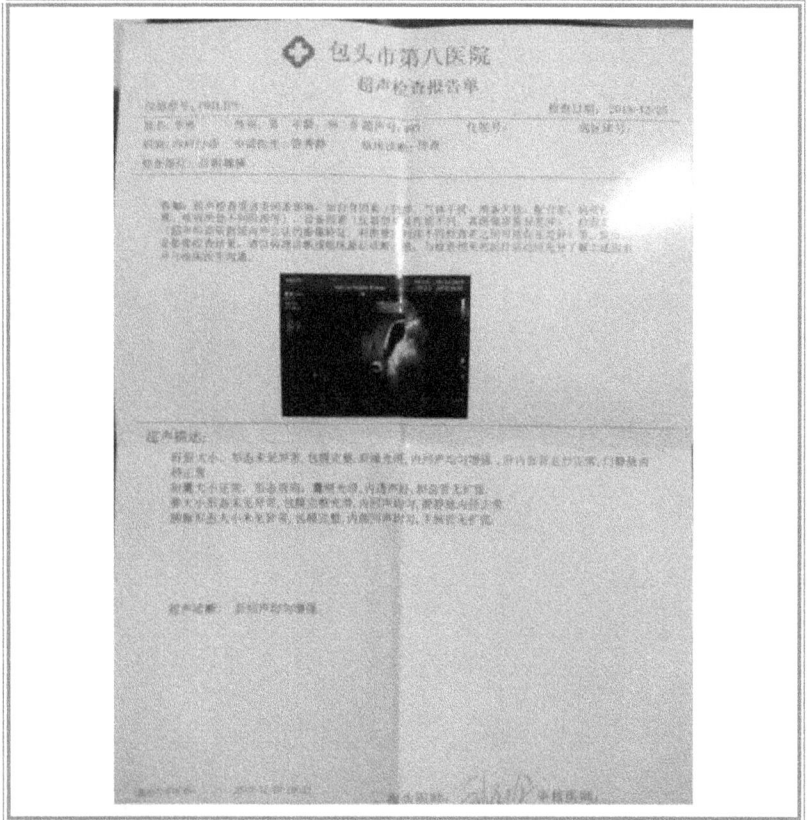

Comments

Yong Li represents a group of people in high risks who feel good about themselves. These people almost never get sick, but if they get sick then it is serious illness, they can even die from it. They never pay attention to their health because their bodies appear to be healthy. They then waste their 'health', and at last, they become unhealthy. Another type of people who always have slight illness are more likely to live longer, because the physical discomfort reminds them and incentivize them to work towards healthiness. Yong Li is a lucky man who has restored health through the early adjustment, and he will make a career because of the energy.

Obesity

Case 1:

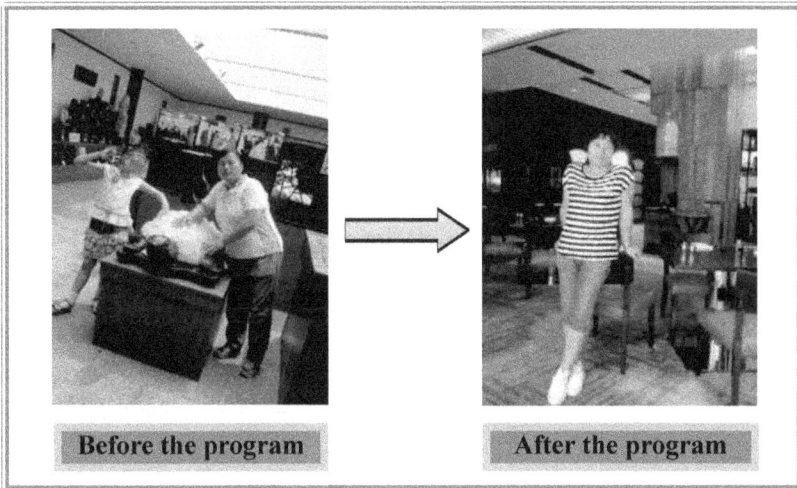

Before the program → After the program

My name is Bingfeng Zhang. I'm from Xinjiang and I live in Jinan now. These are my changes in my physical before and after taking part in Dr. Lu's program.

	Before program	After program
Weight	71KG	61.5KG
BMI	28.1	24.3
Waist size	100CM	76CM
PBPI	110/150	80/115
Fatty liver	Moderate	Mild

I was a Sanda (Chinese Boxing) athlete and had a strong body when I was young. I cannot remember since when did I become big. Everyone who knew me knew that I was not smug. So, after getting fat, I did not think about losing weight at all. I calmly accepted the increasing weight, like how I was indifferent to weather changes.

If it wasn't for a medical examination in 2010, I would still have continued my behaviour, and live with a fat bod every day. These terrible numbers (of the indexes) made me realize for the first time that obesity had brought serious harm to my physical health. I was afraid of the fat on my body when the triglyceride index was increasing, when I had moderate fatty liver and hypertension. I was once healthy, but now because I did not value health, I was no longer healthy. 'No, this is no good', I said to myself. I decided to try to regain my health, so I set my goal and shouted it to my family and friends – 'I want to lose weight!'

In 2010, after using slimming product recommended by my husband's friend, I did not want to lose weight anymore for one whole year. Because the experience of using the slimming products was painful, the memory is still so fresh and I still remember it like yesterday. I had to 5-6 hours out of 24 hours every day in the bathroom, and I had to drink 3L of water, that's why I remember it now. Yet, I knew that losing weight was not easy, so I had to tolerate the pain. Until one day, when I was weak and had no power in my legs and fell onto the floor at home. My husband came and said to me, 'Let's stop this.' That became my excuse of not trying to lose weight. Just like this, for half month of hectic weight loss experience was over because my husband's words.

In 2011, I tried to lose weight again. This time I took a diet. I didn't eat anything every afternoon, but it didn't make any difference to my weight. The only thing it brought every day was hunger and hunger, it was strange. However, I was not going to give up and I chose another method—running. Running was easy for me. I ran 5km every day for half month and reduced 3kg. Yet, to continue it was the hard part. I was panting and sweating every day, while other people were enjoying their lives. The saddest part was that after half a month, no matter how much I ran, I did not lose any more weight. Therefore, I gave up again.

In 2013, I was still trying to lose weight. I used this type of weight loss product. During this process, I could not eat meat and I had to drink more than 8 litres of water every day. It was awful. Although water is the source of life, I still hated it. This type of experience is not something that everyone would have. After bearing such pain for one month, there was no change in my weight so I gave up again.

April 2013 was when I first found out about Dr. Lu program. I went to the training camp with curiosity and hopes, but also with doubts. After all, I tried so many ways but they all failed. My magical pilgrimage started on April 20th. On this day, I ate beef, vegetables, and fruits. I did not eat any staple food and drank about 3L of water. I did some simple aerobics with other guys, 15 minutes each time and twice a day. With this way, my weight changed from 71kg to 69.1kg in just one day. What a surprise! It was wonderful that I had lost 1.9kg without tiring exercises and hunger, at that time I told myself that I must stick to it, this way must be effective.

After the training camp, I formally started implementing the 42-day-short-term program. On the second day of implementation, I stopped taking antihypertensive drugs which I had been taking for over two years. 42 days later, my weight was 61.6kg. I was so excited because it was the first time that the figure of my weight started with 6. Yet, I wanted to know how well my health was, not just weight loss. I took a B-scam ultrasonography and a Comprehensive Metabolic Panel. The data were all normal. In addition to these, since June 4th, 2013, to now, it has been three months, and I have lost another 4.5kg, and my current weight is 57kg. Do you know why? Because Dr. Lu scheme not only helped me to solve the obesity problems, which had been with me for years, and health problems, also it also let me be able to fully grasp the keys of a healthy diet in the 42 days. This is the key to my continued weight loss after adjustment. I believe that I will never be fat again and will continue to be more and more beautiful and confident.

Comments:

Ms. Zhang did not do any strenuous exercise during this process, but she has a better weight loss effect than ever. Why? Strenuous exercise uses the amount of exercise itself to burn fat. Research shows that running 10km increases the energy consumption by around 500 to 700 kilojoules. For every 9 kilojoules, 1 gram of fat is burnt. So, running 10km burns 56 grams to 78 grams of fat. After one month of running 10km every day, only 2.5 to 5 kilograms would be lost. In addition, weight loss by exercising requires continuous exercise for at least 30 minutes, because fat only starts burning after 30 minutes. Exercises that last for less than 30 minutes have no contribution to weight loss. Actually, none of these theories apply to us. The program uses 15 minutes+ of walking or workout program. We are not trying burn fat with excursing, but rather we are trying to improve the metabolic functions, restore the correct energy path, and assist in the sending of fats to all cells throughout the body. This means that the fat stored in the body replace the energy from the stable food consumed. The fats constantly provide energy for 100 trillion cells. Each cell consumes a bit of fat, in one day, the cells consume 0.25 to 0.5 kg of fat in total, that is, 5 to 15 kg of fat in one month. After the short-term program, most people can maintain their weight at the maintenance stage because they develop the right lifestyle. There is also a small portion of people who continue to lose weight after the program, such as Ms. Zhang. There are two reasons: one is the cells are fully activated, so people are often energetic. The other reason is an increase in muscle percentage. Energy, fat and muscle are like light, wax, and core of a candle respectively. The thicker the candle core, the brighter the candle and the more wax burnt. When these people enter the maintenance stage, more energy is burnt than the energy consumed from food. Thus, they continue to lose weight .

Case 2:

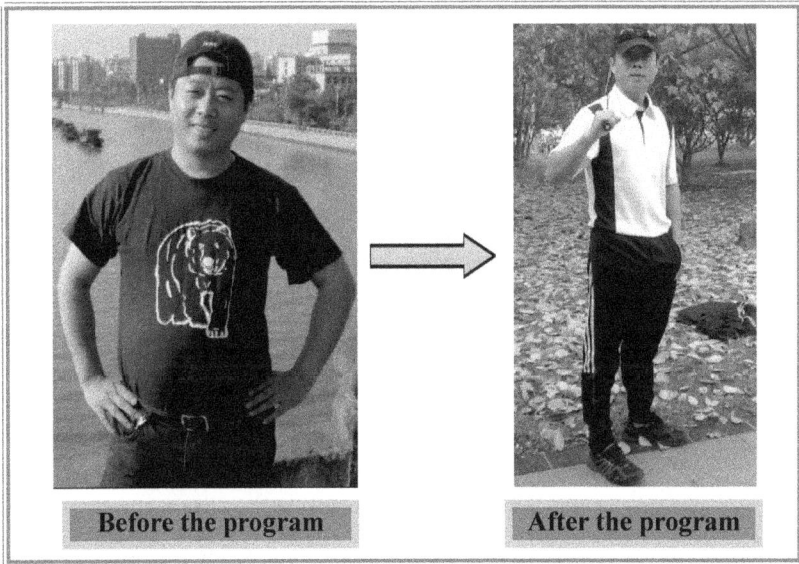

| Before the program | After the program |

My name is Dongsheng Wang. I am from Shanghai, below are my physical statistics before and after I took part in Doctor Lu's program.

	Before program	After program
Weight	83kg	70kg
BMI	27.7	23.4
Waist size	93cm	80cm
Total cholesterol	6.02	3.18

Before program, except the total cholesterol was slightly high, the other indexes were very good. I had always thought that I was very healthy, except for cervical problem, which brought me the problem of hand numbness from time to time. But from the beginning of 2010, I started to hate my big belly. I liked exercising, running, and hiking, however the burden became bigger as the stomach became bigger. I used to run more 10km every night, I didn't feel much before. Yet, after I gained weight the burden became bigger. Early in 2011, my first long run resulted in knee damage, and my doctor forbade me to do the following:

1. lose weight; 2. running was not allowed in the next 3 months. Those who don't run often might not understand, but to me who loves running a lot, this was really painful as I could not participate in the marathons held in Hangzhou, Shanghai and other places, and great pleasure in life was lost. In June 2011, under a friend's recommendation, I participated in Dr. Lu's program, and I began to have a lot of hope. I looked forward to wear my quick-dry shirts and pants early and continue my running life. I was anxious during that time, but when I found my weight gradually declined and my stomach was slowly shrinking, I had the feeling that I would not have to wait for a long time to start running marathons again. After 42 days of short-term intensive program, it surprised me when I stepped on the scale, my weight went back to the number six or seven years ago - 70kg, it was really incredible. Most importantly, I could easily adapt to the program. I did not feel hungry at all. Whenever I did feel hungry, I ate some snacks. I could also eat beef, vegetables and such. I wasn't being tough on my stomach, I ate anything I wanted to. In the course of the process, my mental state was also excellent. At that time, I had the idea that I must thank my friend who let me get rid of the excess body fat under an easy condition, and even the hand numbness caused by the cervical spine, which had troubled me for many years, also recovered. Two years have passed since the program, my basic weight is maintained at about 70kg, and my life is back on track. These changes really let me feel like I am a new person; the program let me regain the happiness from running.

Comments:

The phenomenon of not feeling hungry (like Mr. Wang) during the entire program is very common and normal. Why do people always feel hungry when they're losing weight from diets, whereas this plan doesn't bring hunger? The true cause for hunger is the lack of nutrition in cells. Sometimes the stomach is too full, but one may still feel hungry, that is because the cells are not eating enough. Sometimes the blood sugar is already high, but the person is still hungry, that is because the cells need energy. If you ate meat every day, you would crave for vegetables and rice, because the cells need vitamins. If you ate vegetables every day, you would crave meat, because of cells are lacking protein. This program does not cause hunger because the cells are not lacking nutrition. Where does the nutrition come from? It is from the diet. In addition to the staple food, people also consume meat and vegetables. Moreover, it is from the fat stored in the body, energy conversion will send the body fat to cells, and provide energy, this means that the fats play the roles of staple food.

Case 3:

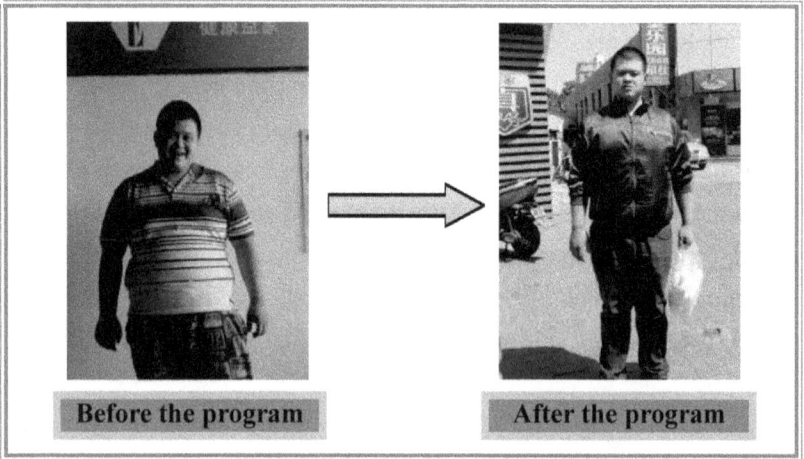

| Before the program | After the program |

My name is Hongyu Liu (son of case 5, disease category, Zhigang Liu). I was born on November 25, 1995. I joined the army at the end of 2012, now I am a ground solider in Beijing Air Force. Being a soldier had been my dream since childhood, but people who were familiar with me knew that it was impossible, because I was so fat that the word 'running' did not relate to me in any way. One year before becoming a soldier, my weight reached a record high of 145 kilos. I could only walk slowly, let alone running. Because of obesity, wherever I went, people would look strangely at me, they discriminated against me, and called me names. So, I was very ashamed to meet people, and lost confidence and felt depressed. I gave up on myself. For various reasons, I dropped out of school, and my dream of being a solider was also crashed.

However, doom did not end just because I was away from my classmates and friends' sarcasm. I started a long weight loss journey. Some of my friends with the same experience told me a famous saying in this circle: weight loss is a lifetime thing. Did weight loss really take a lifetime? I tried a variety of weight loss methods, but all the weight loss programs had one core principle, that was, decline in physical ability, continuous rebound, and the result was that my weight increased from 110kg to 147.5kg during the winter holiday. At that time, the decline in my physical ability was extreme, and my waist size reached 141.6cm, legs around 90cm. At that time what I thought most about was what kind of (army) uniform would fit my body? As a result of weight loss, I sweated when I moved due to physically weakness, and I smelt nasty because of sweat all the time. Every day I only ate, slept, played games, I was incapable of helping my parents to take care of the business. My family felt sorry and helpless for me. I was pessimistic because of the complaints from relatives. As a result, I become depressed. With the increase of the physical burden, fatty liver, heart disease also followed, I didn't know what my future would be, let alone the idea of the future, and the vision of life.

In May 2012, I greeted my life's first turning point. By chance, I got to know Dr. Lu's program, and it let me fundamentally recognize the causes of obesity, as well as its harms to the body. My families tried the program for a month and followed the instructions strictly. The results were pleasing, and I was surprised when I found out that I had successfully and safely reduced 40 kilos, and my physical strength was also greatly enhanced. In order to exercise, I participated in badminton, one hour every session. At the start, I had to take a break every ten minutes. At the end, I only had to take one break for every game I played. From passive defence and shuttlecock picking, to active attacks. Gradually, I started to win games. It made me happy and I regained my confidence. I shared my own experience many times in the training camp, facing the admiration coming from people's eyes, and warm applause. I continued and lost 53kg in total. Fatty liver, myocarditis, heart rhythm all returned to normal. At this time, my dream that had been oppressed for a long time was back again. In order to achieve the dream, I insisted on physical exercise. In November, I returned to my hometown to participate in the new solider registration of year 2013. Hard work paid off. I successfully passed the complex and tedious physical examination, and successfully got enrolled, which made my dream come true.

Now I have been through a year of troops training. I have learned all kinds of military skills. Under the influence of my comrades, I decided to regain the deserted youth. I discussed with my parents and decided to study from the beginning of middle and high school curriculum, and I was determined to enter the military school, to make up for my lost.

It is gratifying that my father saw my changes and had me as his role model. He participated in this plan. His weight was more than 150kg. He also suffered from diabetes and had been taking hypoglycaemic drugs for more than 5 years. After less than six months of implementation, he lost 30kg, all the hypoglycaemic drugs were stopped, and the blood sugar was maintained at a very standard level. This is a very exciting news, and it is Dr. Lu's program that has changed the fate of our family, in which I sincerely thank the things that the plan has done for us. At the same time, we are willing to do our best to promote this project.

The right health guide has fulfilled the dream of my life. Without this adventure, I would still be an obese people, who hated everything, and I would be immersed in my own sadness without doing anything. In the future, I will actively cooperate with the program, cherish the return of this program, and manage my own way of life - stay away from disease and live healthily. This is the inspiration for one year's short experience, and I hope we can help more people with the same needs.

Comments:

Hongyu Liu lost his weight quickly. Many people might ask, 'Isn't it a bit too fast?

The so-called 'experts' often say: 'fat needs to be reduced slowly to keep healthy.' But the question is, why is it unhealthy when it is too fast? How many cases are they for those who have lost weight fast and have become unhealthy? If there are examples, is it the problem of the speed or the actual method? There are so-called 'authorities' who have pointed out that: losing 2-4kg per month is healthy, and not easy to rebound. The question is, where do we get the standard of 2-4kg from? If we lose more than this, why will it affect health? Can the effect be resolved? Why does losing weight too fast bad too fast cause in rebound? Is it the question of too fast or the question of the method? These are no answers, or no one even thinks of the question seriously, or still do not know the answer after thinking.

Speed is relative. Not relative to age, height, or weight, but to one's own metabolic function. If the weight loss was more than the metabolic capacity, then it was fast; vice versa. The standard of the practice is very simple, the more uncomfortable the body feels, it is too fast; vice versa.

The rate of weight loss in this program can be physically controlled. The same program applied to different people had different speeds. In general, the greater the amount of muscle, the faster the speed will be. Energy conversion is to send the fat to the tissue cells, mainly the body muscle cells. Large muscle is like a candle wick, burning fast is like having a bigger wick. Fat gets sent to the cells, if the cells are consumed fast, more fat is sent, and if the consumption is slow, less fat is sent. Thus, the speed of weight loss is controlled by the total demand of 100 trillion cells in the body. Another rule is the younger and the healthier the patient, the faster the weight loss; the unhealthier and older people are not able to lose weight quickly even if they want to. Because when the cells are younger and active, the metabolism is stronger, and the faster the consumption of reserve fat is.

There is also a phenomenon of which that people who lose weight faster are more fit, and their bodies recover faster. Because the faster the speed, the more waste is turned into wealth, and cells receive more energy, accelerating the process of self-repair and reconstruction, so the body improves faster.

Case 4:

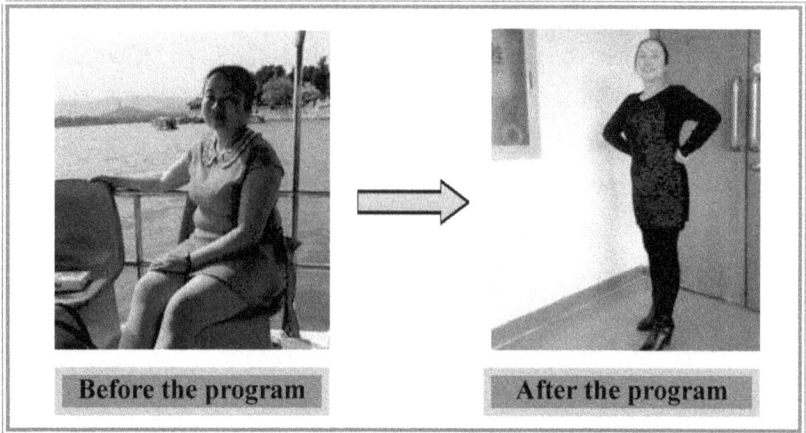

	Before program	After program
Weight	68kg	55kg
BMI	28.1	24.3
Waist size	90cm	73.3cm
Endocrine	Severe disorder	Normal
Fatty liver	Severe	Normal

My name is Ying Wen (wife of case 7, disease category, Jian Wu; mother of case 13, obesity category, Qianlingfang Wu). I am aged 45 years, from Guizhou, now living in Beijing. Below are the data before and after I took part in the Dr. Lu's program:

Hi guys! I am very happy to have such a precious opportunity to share my wonderful experience of weight loss and improving physical chronic disease. My experience was the same as many women. Since giving birth to my daughter, my stomach had become like a tire. I was 160cm, but with a weight of 69.5kg. I was bloated, and I didn't have time to adjust my physical condition as I had been worked as a business executive. The high-intensity work drained all of my energy, so as that when I reached my forties; I felt fatigue both physically and mentally. A variety of chronic diseases also followed. I sought for medical advice everywhere, and bought health care products from a dozen of big companies, but the final effects were minimal. I went to some well-known health examination centre for physical check-ups. My body age made me gasp – 68 years old! I could no longer imagine the future of my life.

At the end of last year, through the introduction of friends, my daughter and I participated in Doctor Lu's program. Before the program, I weighed 68kg, and my sleeping quality was very bad, I also had serious gynaecological disease. My daughter's weight was 81kg (height was 1.64 meters), with bad endocrine, dysmenorrhea, and poor sleeping quality.

After implementation for a week, I lost 3kg. The belly became tighter, and the waist began to show, the facial skin began to tighten up, I felt like I had a small face, which greatly increased my confidence. In addition, signs of improvement of chronic diseases, such as headache, nausea, chest tightness, weak legs, and sleepy, also showed. These symptoms, with the upgrade of energy, also disappeared slowly. Now I work 10 hours every day without feeling tired, even people who are in their twenties or thirties don't have the energy like me. What's more is that I kept asking the coach questions, and gradually, I mastered the formation of Triple H, diabetes, obesity, and how to adjust these problems without rebound. Now, I have lost weight and improved chronic diseases successfully. My daughter also reduced weight from 81kg to 60kg, and she is very happy. Now I have devoted all my time to the cause of 'Giving 100 Million Families a Right Way of Living and Keeping Them Away from The Triple H and Obesity' businesses. This career has given me a sense of mission and responsibility. I am willing to put in all my time and effort to make the world more beautiful!

Case 5:

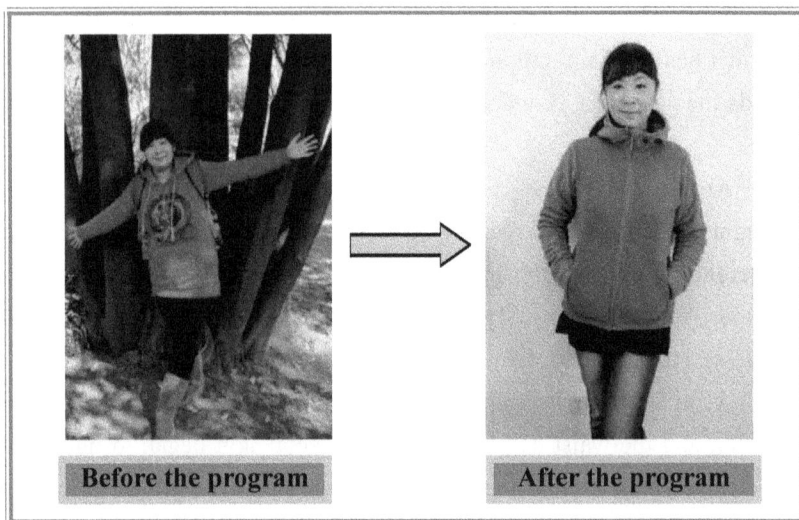

| Before the program | After the program |

My name is Chunxue Yang, from Yunnan, now living in Kunming. My physical data before and after participating in Dr. Lu program are as below:

	Before program	After program
Weight	73kg	59kg
BMI	28.1	24.3
Waist size	103.3cm	76.6cm

I participated in the Lu's program by chance. Before that, I had been fat for more than ten years. The highest record reached 75kg. Although

	Before program	After program
Weight	73kg	59kg
BMI	28.1	24.3
Waist size	103.3cm	76.6cm

On May 30, 2012, I started a short-term intensive program that lasted for two cycles to reduce weight, and I strictly followed my coach's menu. On September 6, after a short time of two cycles, my weight reduced from 73kg to 59kg, a total weight loss of 14kg, waist size reduced from

103.3cm to 76.6cm. Notably, my blood pressure also went down. After getting tested, the excessive visceral fat also returned to normal, and my face colour turned better. I look younger, and climbing the stairs is not as tiring as before. The happiest thing is that a lot of friends ask when they meet me, 'Woe, how have you become so skinning after a few months?' I am really happy and I can wear beautiful clothes again.

Case 6:

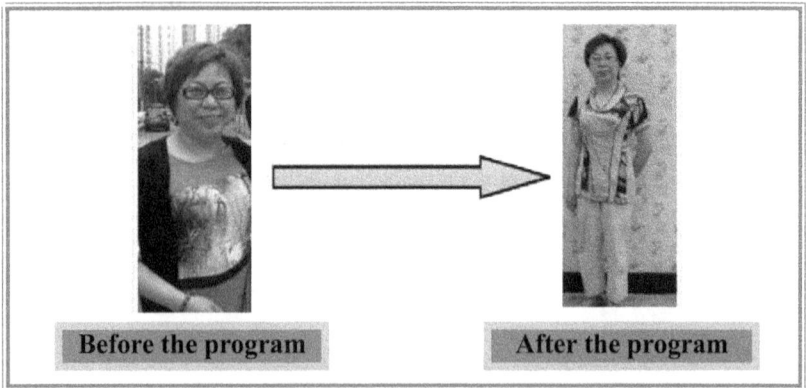

| Before the program | After the program |

My name is Yongna Pei, 47 years old, general manager of an equipment company. I was recommended by my classmates in university, and on March 29th, 2013, I participated in Beijing's training camp activities, and began to use Dr. Lu's adjustment program. At the end of a short-term program, I reduced 9kg easily, and I had a perfect body shape. I went back to Beijing with the changes and began to explore the new adjustment plan and idea.

I had typical metabolic disorder, and I gained fat even I ate less. When I was young, I had a good body shape, but in the last two years, my body became fat and bloated. With a fat body, it was difficult to buy clothes. When there were people around or were talking body shapes, I always felt very embarrassed. Facing this situation, I thought of losing weight many times, but the thought of weight loss and the side effects of rebound stopped my thinking.

This program is different from the traditional weight loss method. Through diet adjustment, based on science, with simple adjustment process, satisfactory effects, it does not have any side effects to the body. After a cycle of adjustment, my body was restored, and the metabolic capacity of each organ was also restored. I think the formation of this program contributes significantly to the mankind!

Dr. Lu's program is really the gospel for obese people! My personal experience made me believe that it can help countless people. So I have begun to share around the circle of friends, and just five months' time, I got 100 people to implement this program.

Watching more and more friends restore their beautiful bodies, get rid of Triple H drugs, and disappearance of sub-health state, I felt happy from the heart. At the same time, I admire the R & D team of this program from the core, and people who promoted this program at the beginning! I will promote with heart, so that more people can understand the programed benefit!

Case 7:

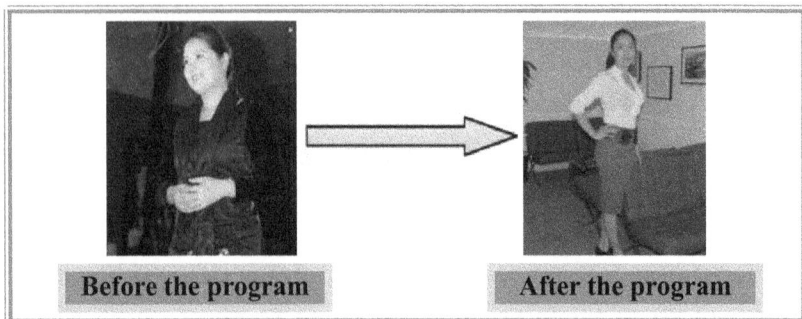

| Before the program | After the program |

My name is Jing Wu (sister of case 6, disease category, Mei Wu). I knew that many weight loss programs had side effects on the body, so I dared not lose weight blindly. Because after weight loss, the body would become weak, and finally it would rebound, leaving me with an unhealthy body. So, I did not care much about my fat body shape. Yet, with the increase in age, my energy gradually decreased, and the skin was loosened. I wanted to start metabolism adjustment, but I was not able to find a good way. After seeing the changes of my sister, I decided to carry out metabolic adjustment. Under the strict supervision of my sister, I had a good experience. In the second week, my body changed a lot, it was not only energetic, but my mental state was good, and my skin was tight. Before, the morning alarm clock would continue to alert for one hour until I woke up, and now I want to get up with a simple turn of my body. I lost more than 5kg, and all organs have been repaired. For a whole course, I felt relaxed, I reduced a lot of fat and the problems that I did not think of were also solved. It was really an unexpected surprise.

Because I experienced it myself, and received good effects, and the operation of this program is simple, I am very optimistic about its prospects, and I have included this program in my career. Although it is just at its beginning, my progress is not big, in previous years, tens of thousands of successful cases have proved its effects, and I believe I will be able to promote it well.

Case 8:

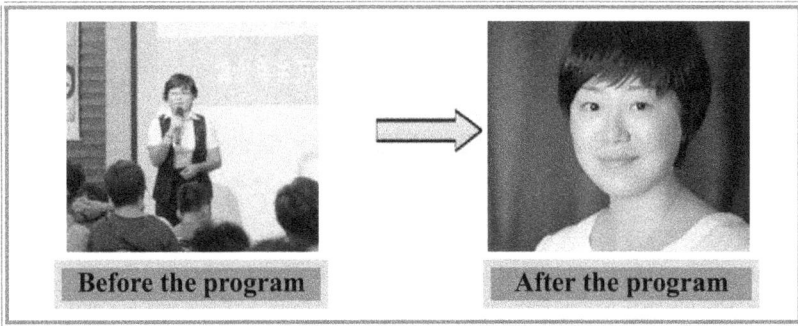

Before the program → After the program

My name is Liangliang Zhang, a senior manager of a bank in Guangzhou. I have a happy family, my husband loves me, and my daughter is also well-behaved, and I have a decent job. I should feel happy for all this. But it was not the case, there was a problem which bugged me for a long time, which was my weight problem. I was less than 1.6m in height, but weighted 63kg, and I looked swollen, the baby fat face often made me sigh when I looked into the mirror.

I am a northerner. I was only around 50kg when I first arrived at Guangzhou and with a more fit figure. But after settled here, I was not used to the environment here, because of my work, I had a lot of dinners outside, and the diet was not regular. The main reason was overeating, and uncontrolled consumption of snacks. So, after a few years, my weight also slowly went up with these bad habits, when I realized it, it was too late. I had also tried a lot of weight loss methods, but the result was that the weight I lost was regained.

Obesity brought me not only body changes and a chubby face, also the degradation of body functions, and I easily became tired, also with a pale face. I looked much older than my actual age. God! If I kept going like this, would I suffer from Triple H (high blood pressure, high blood lipids, and high blood sugar)?

However, after I used one cycle of Dr. Lu's program, I was surprised to find that my baby fat was gone, and I felt relaxed, the body functions were restored, even my mother said I looked ten years younger. Listening to what she said, I knew I had made a right choice.

This program gave me a comfortable feeling. For 42 days of the short-term treatment, I reduced from 63kg to 55kg, although I didn't reach my original weight before I came to the South, I was quite satisfied. My body had been improved all around, and the whole process was relatively easy. Previously I tried some drugs to lose weight, although they did work towards lose weight, but the process was very hard and miserable, and the weight rebounded again.

Comfort is a major feature of this adjustment program, and during the adjustment process, it gave me the feeling that I could lose weight without diet. Every day I ate fruits and vegetables, and I could also eat beef, chicken. When you were hungry you could eat small snacks. I had never tried eating when hungry in other methods.

I remembered the beginning of the adjustment, symptoms of coughing appeared for several days. I asked the coach (during adjustment, there is an appointed coach to track your whole process) my problems, he told me that this was because my lungs were not good since I was a child, and it was the result of long-term use of antibiotics. I did what the coach told me and through adjustment, the body functions really recovered.

After the program, I found my swollen body had become light and tight, I felt like the excess water in the body was gone, and the skin had become rosy, full of flexibility, I am full of energy. I also want to tell you a secret that this adjustment program will not let the breasts become small. After program, I think my chest is more tight and elastic than before.

Since the adjustment, I can wear the clothes that I dare not wear previously, and I can finally say goodbye to my XXL banking uniform. Many of my friends and colleagues saw my recent changes, all came to learn from me, and asked me how I can make such a big change within a short time of one month. I felt like I was a different person with more energy and much younger.

Since I successfully lost weight, my husband loves me more, and it makes me feel very good. Although he also treated me nice before, but never like this! Anyway, since the adjusted in accordance with the program, I feel my world is full of sunshine, it feels good!

Case 9:

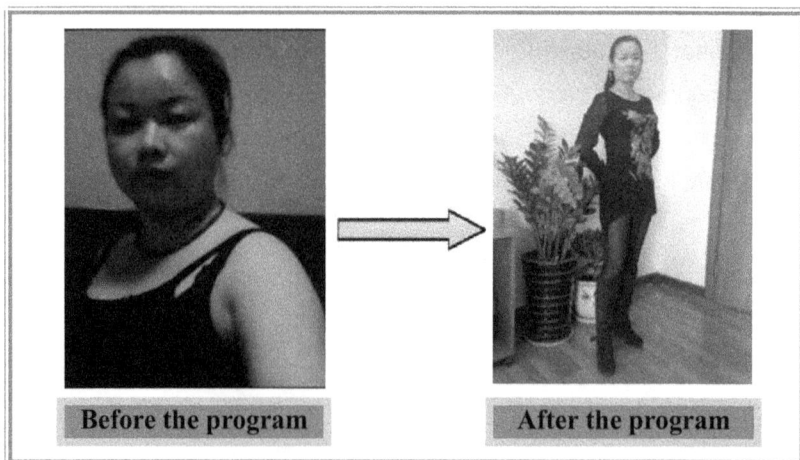

| Before the program | After the program |

Hello everyone! I am Wenjing Ye, from Qingdao, Shandong. Before using this program, my weight reached 79kg, waist size was 90cm. After 42 days of short-term program, my weight reduced to 65kg, waist size was 76.6cm. Within a month's time, Dr. Lu's program allowed me to throw away many large -sized clothes and put on XL clothes of my dreams, and regain self-confidence.

Because I had been working outside for in recent years, I had an irregular lifestyle. This led to endocrine disorders, and my body went out of shape. I used a variety of weight loss methods. Because of the ingredients taken in from oral administration (from weight losing medication), my heart beat sometimes accelerated all a sudden, with intense suffocation. I wasn't dared to continue using it, so the method failed. However, I was still trying find a good way to lose weight.

By chance, I meet a coach from Dr. Lu's program. After in-depth learning, I understood that the program was not simply using medication to adjust body conditions. Rather, the program used scientific diet plans and changed incorrect lifestyles. In particular, I heard that I did not need to do strenuous exercise, but also I did not have to starve. I could eat chicken, duck, fish, beef, beans, eggs, milk, fruit, and vegetables. Apparently. I could reduce 2 to 3 kg every week. I was dying to try it out. After a week's time, the magic happened to my body, which verified the truth. I lost 4kg in one week, and in 42 days' time, I lost 14kg in total! The biggest surprise was not only this, but 'creaky knees', that had accompanied me for years, disappeared. After 6 months, I didn't feel uncomfortable, and my body shape was maintained well.

Friends around me were very shocked about my changes, and also participated in the program to change their lifestyles. Ms. Wen began to implement the program with her family. Her daughter was a little fat girl, she lost 20kg in two months. Her husband's belly disappeared, his legs didn't hurt anymore. This let us see the future of this course, the program will expand to a big one. Because we are surrounded by many Triple H people, so Ms. Wen, several friends and I joined the industry without hesitation, hoping to help more obese and Triple H people to find self-confidence, and become healthy again!

Comments:

The above cases are weight loss, with good body shaping effects. Their weight loss can be roughly summarized into three points:

Body Shaping: the most obvious is waist shaping, because the program is mainly countering insulin resistance. One of the signs of insulin resistance is waist thickening, when the energy path is corrected, insulin resistance is eliminated, so waist size becomes smaller. In addition to the waist, the shoulder, back, legs, buttocks will also reduce fat. The parts, which have more fat, have more obvious fat reduction.

Skin Tightening: we have found that during the program, the skin on the chest, face and bottom, have tightened. Because this program does not reduce the protein, it also turns waste into wealth. It speeds up the repair of subcutaneous protein and dermis. So, the skin becomes tighter and the wrinkles are reduced.

Skin Tone Improvement: during the program, the improved skin colour phenomenon is very common. There are two main reasons, one is that the program removes intestinal toxins. After the elimination of intestinal toxins, acnes and spots can be significantly improved; the second is there is more blood. When the blood is sufficient, skin will be glowing and rosy. Health and beauty can both be gained, and we can even say that only the internal health can bring the external glory, investing in health is investing in beauty.

Case 10

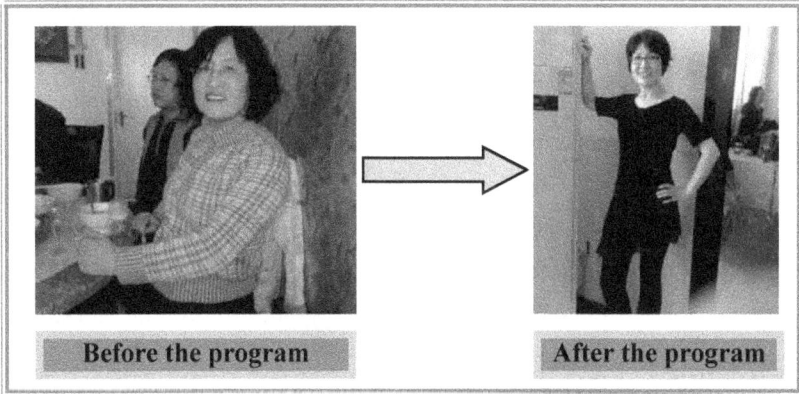

Before the program → After the program

My name is Mingyue Liu, 48 years old, a practicing pharmacist. I implemented the short-term intensive program from July 7, 2012 to August 24. I was 61kg before the program, afterwards, I weighed 51kg, a weight loss of 10kg. Before the program, my waist size was 78.3cm, after the program was 70cm, my waist size reduced by 8.3cm.

I will tell you about my adjustment experience. Before program, there was an accumulation of fat in my abdomen. When I tried to squat, it was very inconvenient. I had loosened limb muscles, and often felt sleepy and lazy, I had no energy every day. I had difficulties to fall asleep, and it was difficult to fall sleep again after waking up at night. I bad sleeping quality, constipation, freckles, breast swelling before menstrual, lethargy and other symptoms. In June 2012, I went to Shanxi Provincial People's Hospital and did a thorough Comprehensive Metabolic Panel, and all indicators were normal. After one short-term adjustment plan, plus a week of just fruit and vegetable juice, the magic effect appeared. Friends who met me said I looked like another person: the skin was tight, rosy, and the sports faded. I looked a lot smaller overall. I looked more energetic, and younger, yet they had only seen my external changes, in fact, changes in the body were the most important. The quality of sleep greatly improved, I could fall asleep easily and I would not wake up at night. I was refreshed in the morning, I was energetic every day and constipation problems were solved. My happiness and satisfaction were shown through my facial expressions. I wear beautiful clothes every day to visit friends and wanted to show all the beautiful things to them.

With such good method and good effects, I must promote it.

The program combines the concept of Chinese medicine treatment, Western nutrition, human physiology and other characteristics. The program is reasonable and has a theory. As a health worker (26 years being a pharmaceutical engineer), it is my duty to promote good health concepts and methods.

As a disciple of Buddhism, I am willing to spread wisdom to the public, help more people to build the right way of living, keep them away from chronic diseases, reduce or even get rid of drug dependence and improve the quality of life. I like to bring knowledge to others, bring others health, and I enjoy the happiness after I helped people.

When reaching middle age, I have finally found my favourite and more suitable career, I can use what I have learned during these years to help people and enjoy it. I have decided I will not change my goal. Including the course in my future life, for the cause of human health, I will contribute as much as I can.

Comments:

Ms. Liu is both the beneficiary of the program and the promoters of the program. Using lifestyle to solve lifestyle disease is a huge project of the generation; it needs a team to do the project. What is the most important trait of this team? From our point of view, it is love. So where does the love come from? We think the easiest way to have love is to experience. Through the emotional experience, coupled with the theoretical study, one will have burning passion and love. Caring people have a great influence to the world, because they burn themselves to illuminate others, and even ignite others, and finally illuminate the world.

Case 11:

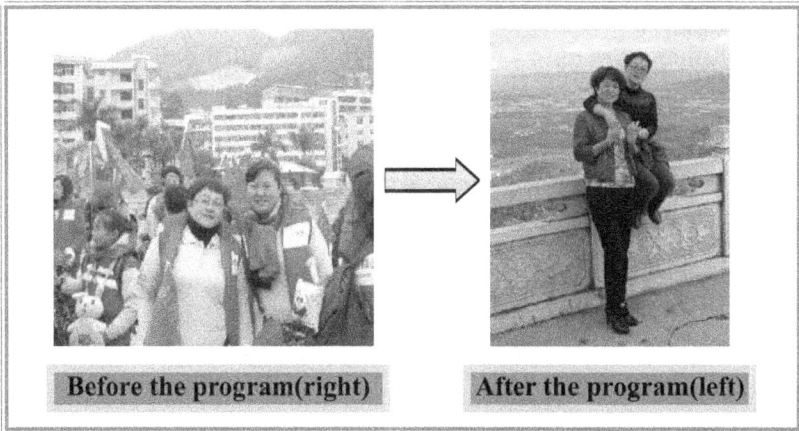

Before the program(right) | After the program(left)

My name is Jing Sun, female, 43 years old, from Yunnan Chuxiong, engaged in the medical industry. Before weight loss, I weighed 66kg, waist size was 91.6cm, and I had 49,000 platelets. After weight loss, I weighed 58kg, waist size was 73.3cm, and had 79,000 platelets.

I have always been passionate about life, I also love outdoor sports, and I walk every day, I always climb mountains. I didn't allow myself to be lazy because I think as long as we move, we would be healthy. I got the habit of exercising from my father. He is 80 years old now. His body is very strong, all healthy physical examination indicators are normal. Therefore, I only focused on the importance of sports to health, but ignored diet habits and other factors.

Over the years, I had not realized that bad eating habits would bring harm to the family. I felt very healthy, but my son gained weight every day, so I felt very worried and I thought I was doing something wrong. My son was only 15 years old, but he weighed 108kg, and we could not find the cause. We thought that he was eating too much, and did not exercise enough, so we asked him to increase the amount of exercise. Yet, forced to exercise was too painful for him, he did not want to exercise. Looking at how much pain he was in, I backed off. This become a cause for conflicts and arguments in our family, it affected the family's normal atmosphere. Because of obesity, my son's study was also affected. My husband and I learnt medicine back at school, and came up many loss methods, but did not dare to let our son to try. We were afraid that blind weight loss would bring bad influence on the body, but we still thought that something had been missing and we were very worried.

Until one day my friend told me that there was a healthy way to lose weight. You could easily lose weight, but also eat. I was sceptical. Nowadays weight loss was about diet or exercise, drugs or technology, and with side effects. Thinking of these, I did not believe it immediately, and I did not see her when she was in her weight losing period. A month has passed, my friend suddenly appeared, and surprised me, she turned from a fat girl to a slim beauty! Her mental state was much better than before, full of vitality. I could not believe my eyes, that moment, I seemed to be able to see my son become healthy, so my first thought was to let him participate in this program.

At the beginning, my son was not to it, because he used to high fat and high carbohydrate diet, and could not continue. He protested, but under coach's patient explanation and guidance, he still continued because he felt the pleasure weight loss had brought at the beginning. In one week, my son lost 6kg. At the end of a short-term program (42 days), he successfully lost 12kg. My son was so happy, he felt his body became lighter, belly was smaller, more energetic, and better temper. Unfortunately, when the holiday ended, he went back to boarding school. Due to limited choices of food and study pressure, he had to stop temporarily. Yet he was very confident that he would continue the program after school finished, he wanted to make himself as tall and straight and handsome as other student.

My fat reduction effects were also good. I was a thrombocytopenic purpura patient before for more than 20 years. I took pills all the time, damaging the liver, but still, I could not stop. Even though my husband

and I were doctors, we could not do anything. Before fat reduction, I was worried that this fat reduction program would affect my body, scared of bad influences on my platelets, but the coach said that Dr. Lu's program was to help restoring the instinct of the body, also known as self-healing ability, and it would only bring benefits to my disease. He assured me to take the program, and during weight loss, I stopped my pills, and finished one short cycle.

After a short period of time, I went to hospital to have a check-up, and the results made my husband and me so happy! My platelet actually rose to a level which I had not able to reach even when I took pills. Before, when I was taking pills, my platelets never surpassed 50000. After the program, without pills, and after a period of weight loss, it even reached to 79,000! I felt energetic and younger, and I felt relaxed when exercise. I did not take drugs for platelets; but the body was improving. I did not need to take any pills after weight lost, which was the most obvious effect. I think our family will be away from the drug, and closer and closer to health. Through this opportunity of participating in Dr. Lu's program, it not only let me get healthy, but also let me learn how to live a healthy life, and how to get the right habits. I will always implement the long-term plan, and also encourage friends and family to participate, so that everyone will benefit from it! Images above are taken before and after weight loss for comparison purposes, let us witness the changes together!

Comments:

Ms. Sun's primary thrombocytopenic purpura has improved, but the etiology of such diseases is still unknown. Through the program, platelets reached up to 79,000 without eating pills. Considering it increased from less than 5000 when taking pills, it was a great improvement. Some people may ask, this program helps to adjust metabolism, so for what kinds of problems would this program be useful? The usefulness depends on the genes on one person. If one is born with such functions, then the method would be useful since the method is to restore functions. If one is not born with certain functions, then the method would not be useful because there are no functions to restore.

Case 12

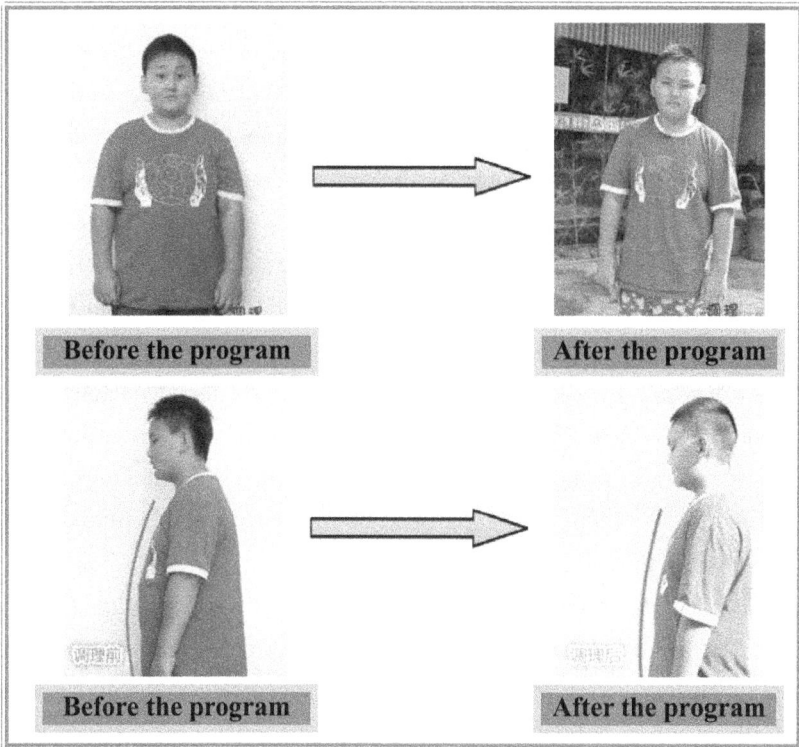

Before the program	After the program

Before the program	After the program

When Jiahao was 7 years old, I divorced with his father, and I lived alone with my son and daughter. Without any source of income, we had done everything to make a living. In the first two to three years, as long as the work made money, I would take it. After several years of hard work, I opened my own restaurant after several years of hard work. Until one day, I found my 10-year-old son weighed 66kg, but without growth in height. I suddenly realized the seriousness of the problem. In the past because of I was busy at work every day, he went to the fast food restaurant to eat high-calorie hamburgers and fried chicken nuggets with the money I gave him. I did not have time to accompany him, so he was always very lonely, and played computer day and night. Because of the lack of exercise, he gained weight. Every time I came back home, he was sound asleep. Then, he became short-tempered. If he felt unhappy, he would roll on the floor and cry.

I learned from school that because of my son is fat, other kids often laughed at him, so he did not play with other students, and was unwilling to participate in class activities. He became more and more introvert. I was busy with business, and did not have enough time to comfort him, until I received the teacher's call. The teacher said that he was bullying classmate. After he came back home I began to teach him, being annoyed by work; I could not control myself and I hit him. My son held the tears back with grief and said, 'Mum, my classmate said that I was born by a pig, and that was why I was this fat! That was why I fought with him! The teacher misunderstood me as I was big!' I cried out loud after listening to what he said! It was my fault and I did not figure out the reason for the fight. Fat people shall not be called pig and they were not born with faults.

I decided to take him to the hospital to have a check-up. The high cholesterol on the results reminded me of how tired he was when he climbed stairs. He was only ten! This was my son we were talking about! Such a young child with such high cholesterol! I was heartbroken. I finally realized that obesity was a disease. It would not only affect him physically, but also mentally as he grew up. As a mother, I did not want my son to live in mockery for the rest of his life.

I felt remorse. Why I did not take good care of my son? Fortunately, there was still a chance to make up. I decided to take my son to lose weight! A lot of beauty salons could help people to lose weight, but they did not dare to take in a ten years old child, mainly because children were still growing, and one mistake would cost the whole body. I started to inquire about success stories about children weight loss, and by chance I learnt, from a beautician friend, that training camp of Dr. Lu was looking for obese volunteer, and I decided to let my son have a try.

Before attending the event, I still had some concerns, because you could not eat fine rice and other refined food during the diet, but they ate a mixture of vegetables, fruits, protein meal. I was worried that it would affect my child's physical development. Yet, after a day of experience Jiahao lost by 1.5kg, and he felt better than the before, so I decided to try it myself too.

In order to give my child a role model, I decided to follow him to improve my body, and ate what he ate. I wanted to use my own unique way to make him continue! This time I would not let him to face it alone, this was the only thing I could do for him! School teachers began to question my practice, but after understanding that this did no harm do the body, and could adjust the body's metabolic orbit, they gave approval. Adjusted a dozen days of nursing, I found the overhung fat on my son's back and neck became smaller, hard fat on the belly turned soft. The coach told me that these were the body signs of a comprehensive adjustment.

The most surprising thing was in the process of weight loss, my son and I had more opportunities to communicate, and his temper and emotions became better. He knew to discuss with me when he has problems and in a politer way. After one cycle, his weight dropped to 60kg, a total weight loss of 6kg, he looked energetic than before. He had stopped short-term intensive program for some time, and there was no sign of rebound. He used to binge eat, but now he had changed to a healthy eating habit.

In the adjustment process I also benefitted. Before the program, every time the menstruation was my 'nightmare. I would vomit and had diarrhoea when I had dysmenorrhea, and had to make injection to ease the symptoms. I could not work normally in this period. In August this year before the program, after taking a B-ultrasound, doctor told me that there were multiple uterine fibroids in the uterus. After implementing the program with my son in October, in early November I went to the hospital for examination, the doctor told me only one fibroids left in the uterus, and it was improving. For as short as one month, my son and I had such a big change, so I really believed that this program was not just to lose weight, but more importantly, it was to help people to be healthy!

Looking at how my son had become healthier and healthier day by day, and seeing the test result once again, I was very pleased! I would like to say to those who are like me, as a mother, the greatest happiness is when she is able to protect her children!

Case 13:

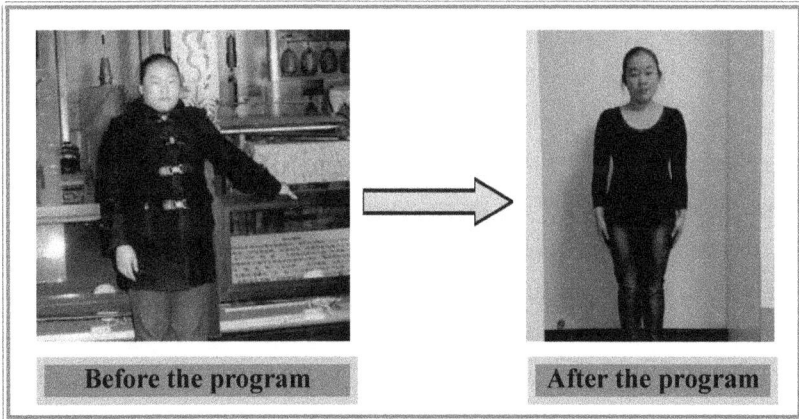

| Before the program | After the program |

I am Qianlinfang Wu (daughter of case 4, obese category, Ying Wen, and case 7, disease category, Jian Wu), from Guizhou, now living in Kaiyang County, Guiyang City. Below is the physical data before and after I took part in Dr. Lu's program:

	Before program	After program
Weight	81kg	60kg
Endocrine disorders	Severe dysmenorrhea	normal
Sleep	sleepless	normal

I am a high school student. I was fat even since I was a child and I did not remember ever being skinny before. As said, a child who had been fat from childhood should be used to obesity, but when I went out to buy clothes I was very hurt. The shop assistant was always rummaging closet after closet and told me that there are no sizes that would suit me. I had tried a lot of weight loss methods, especially this weight loss package. I spent more than twenty thousand yuan (approx. $2750 USD) on this weight loss package, but I only lost 2kg. My mother was furious when she saw such results, and immediately ordered me to give up on losing weight. If I only wanted to lose weight for a better appearance, then it would have been fine to give up. However, although I appeared healthy, I suffered from insomnia, dysmenorrhea, sleepy, which made me very depressed.

Three months ago, my mother came home excitedly ad told me that Ms. Ye lost weight successfully after implementing a special diet program, now her body was quite slim, and it only took two months to achieve such a good result. I was very happy and thought that I would try hard this time, I hoped for losing weight successfully.

I used to lose weight by stop eating food, even if I was hungry, I did not allow myself to eat; but now I could can eat when I was hungry and I could even eat meat. I was very excited, and ate according to the menu. In only one day, my weight fell by a few kilos. It was so wonderful. At the beginning, I was sleepy at noon, but I insisted on once I knew that it was a sign of improvement. Classmates and teachers saw my daily changes, and were very surprised. After class, they gathered around and asked me how I became slimmer and slimmer. I am willing to go to the clothing stores now, and I can buy the clothes that I could not buy before. Now looking into the mirror, the fat me is gone, instead, I am a girl with pale and soft skin. I am so happy.

There is a better surprise to tell you guys! My sleeping quality is now very good, dysmenorrhea has disappeared, and my memory has also become good. My energy is better than others and they are very envious of me. I am now a happy, lucky girl! Thanks to Dr. Lu's program and I will share this program with more friends.

Comments:

Now, many parents will encounter such a problem, they dare not let their children lose weight when the children are obese during adolescence, in fear of that losing weight would influence their growth and development. The reason why a person is fat is because s/he is not healthy. When the body is healthy, weight will naturally fall. The essence of the program is not a weight loss program, but a health plan. It does not reduce nutrition, but rather, it increases nutrition. For example, in the diet of each meal, protein, vitamins, minerals are sufficient. Although there is no staple food, but through energy conversion, the body can transform excess fat into energy and supply those to the cells. So, there are not lack of energy or trace elements, and they are even more sufficient than normal diet. It does not affect the development, but beneficial to development.

The effects of obesity on children during development are disastrous. Because obesity is a metabolic disorder in the body, nutrition cannot be supplied for bone growth and organ development, but to be stored as fat. This has three main problems: 1. Kids are more likely to suffer from Triple H after they grow up; 2. All the development of the body have been affected, not only the bones, as well as sexual organs and the brain, because the raw materials needed for development are not enough; 3. Energy of the kids are affected, resulting in fatigue and learning inefficiency. So children who have obesity should lose weight. This program is not only for weight loss, the essence is the recovery of human metabolism. Only when the metabolism is normal, s/he will not be fat even if s/he eats more than before. Rather, they will grow better, be more energetic, easier to learn with better efficiency. This is because the nutrition is supplied to the cells.

Case 14:

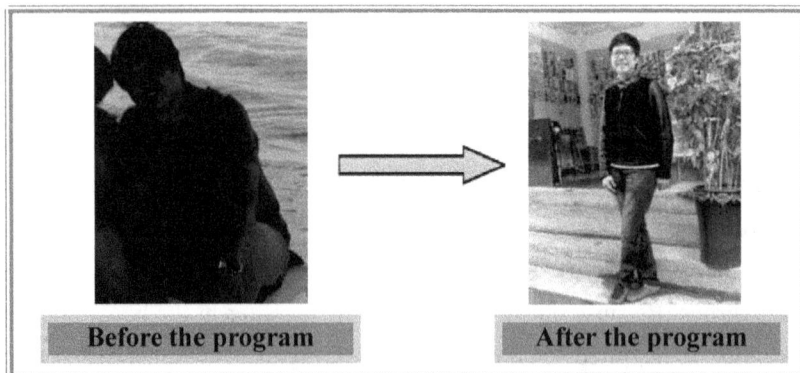

| | Before the program | After the program |

My name is Dan Li. I am from Wuhan, currently living in Kunming, Yunan. Below is my physical data before and after I took part in Doctor Lu's program:

	Before program	After program
Weight	83kg	66kg
Blood glucose	Around 12	Around 6
Waist size	105cm	80cm

The original purpose of participating in Doctor Lu's program was not to lose weight, because when you thought of it, I was already 38 years old, a woman coming to this age, a weight gain was normal. Not to mention that I was 171 cm tall, so although I was fat, but it was not so terrible. During the Chinese New Year in 2011, I was in Kunming First People's Hospital and did a small operation. The operation was very successful, but after the surgery I became melancholy. Because during surgery, the doctor found out my blood sugar was too high, after more than a week of detailed examination, the doctor officially announced to me that I had mild diabetes. Although I did not need to use drugs to control blood sugar, but I must pay attention to the diet in the future, and must take a walk every day after dinner. The most influential sentence was 'It is very unfortunate, you are too young to get this disease.' To tell you the truth, I did not know how serious diabetes was, but when I heard this sentence, I was shocked. Because it seemed like only old people would get this disease. Later, I asked the doctor about how to cure this disease, the doctor gave me two words 'weight loss', and from that time onwards, and I began to think about losing weight.

Of course, I was not so lucky, I did not know Dr. Lu's program at the start. I found a variety of ways to lose weight: eating fruits, capsules, and such. I spent money, and time, but the results were not satisfactory. Until one day, I met a friend who I had not met for 2 months, and I found that she had lost a lot of weight, and she introduced to me Dr. Lu's program. The next day I found a coach through friends for further understanding. On August 3, 2012, I officially began to lose weight. I strictly enforced this program. On September 30, 2012, it had been one and a half cycles, I lost 17kg. I had normal blood sugar and I loosed younger. Until now, it has been over a year since implementing the program, there has not been any rebound. Because I have gotten a healthy diet and living habits through learning and practicing this program. So it is easy to keep. I hope that people like me can participate in the program as early as possible, so they can benefit early.

Comments:

From the end of the intervention till now, almost more than a year has passed and Ms. Li has not rebounded, which is a very common phenomenon. In fact, the program is a combination of short-term long-term and lifelong program. Short-term is the adjustment of metabolism, long-term is the maintenance of metabolism. Lifetime maintenance is a natural continuation of short-term adjustment. Early in the adjustment, a long-term concept needs to be established, and with an intention to form a habit in the beginning, then follow the habit on purpose after it becomes natural. If one only implements short-term adjustment, there is only a period of short-lived health. Only if the long-term habits are established, then it is a healthy life.

Case 15:

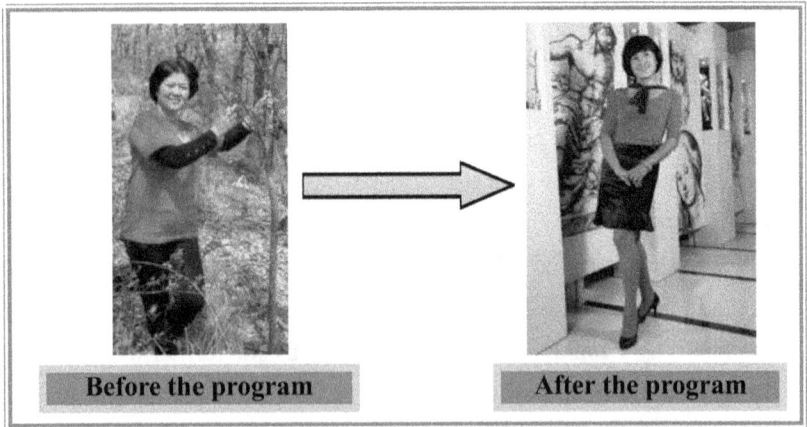

| Before the program | After the program |

I am Yan Yang, female, 50 years old, from Kunming, Yunnan, a doctor. Before weight losses, I weighed 66kg, waist size was 90cm. After weight loss, I weighed 58kg, waist size was 76.6cm. Before and after the program, Comprehensive Metabolic Panel indicators were all in the normal range.

One of the signs of a mature person is to turn the focus away from the external things to themselves. I knew my health changed dramatically after September 2010. Due to additional workload, I suddenly felt everything was not right, so that an ordinary cold can took three months to be cured, so I had to go check in the hospital on January. Although all medical, imaging, Comprehensive Metabolic Panel indicators were in the normal range, but with my own national professional practitioner's qualifications, I understood that I was in sub-health state.

May 22-24, 2011 in Beijing, I participated in the 'The Third Chinese Medical Association Disease Cure Peak Forum', and was attracted by the speech of the last speaker- Dr. Lu, and established a new direction for my career and life.

May 27, I participated in the training camp in Changping, Beijing. The data were: height was 160cm, weight was 66kg, and waist size was

90cm. After 6 weeks of weight loss, my weight was 58kg, waist size was 76.6cm, and my skin became smooth, delicate and glowing, this was the most noticeable change. Yet, these were for others to see, I did not care about these changes that much, because there were more important things that affected me. After the implementation of this program, the most wonderful change in my body was the improvement of sub-health state: haemorrhoids that had troubled me for many years and did not cured after two surgical treatments, disappeared after bleeding on the third day and sixteenth day of adjustment. On the fifth day, cervical spondylosis that would occur suddenly was relieving slowly, and I was no longer troubled by this. Severe dizziness, weak knees, and skin rash on the back and bilateral ribs, all improved on the ninth day, thirteenth day, and seventh day respectively.

Through the study of Dr. Lu's Cell Comprehensive Revitalisation Program, the behavioural health wisdom model, energy path theory, and I had put them into practice. I gradually changed, and cultivated a new correct way of life. My physical conditions got better and better. As I mastered the weight management method, I could adjust my weight according to my will. Also, my body and heart are getting younger.

As the first beneficiary of Doctor Lu's program in Yunnan Province, and as a medical worker, I, with a sense of mission, joined Dr. Lu's team. For more than three years, I have been working for the goal of 'benefiting the public' and set my colleagues as my role models. I try to help others to maintain health, to achieve the value of life, and at the same time, to maximize our values in life.

For more than three years, I've watched the physical and psychological changes in the beneficiaries around me, my heart is filled with comfort and calm. Those little misunderstanding, have already gone with the wind, and I will go on. At the same time, I hope that my classmates and colleagues can quickly change their thinking under the state of rapid growth of Triple H patients, myocardial infarction and other metabolic diseases. Like Dr. Lu, they need to rethink about the 'biomedical model' that has ruled the medical industry for 200 years. I hope that the Government can start a 'New Life' campaign to advocate the correct way of life, that is, to solve lifestyle disease with lifestyle.

Comments:

I met with Dr. Yang face to face, and I could feel her sense of mission and her desire to find the meaning of life, as well as her determination to join in this career for the rest of her life. Solving lifestyle disease with lifestyle is a huge project of this generation. For the expansion of this project, many experts, like Dr. Yang, are needed. First, women are more suitable because women can influence a nation by influencing a family; second, doctors are appropriate for this career, because the public believe in authority; third, the entrepreneurs are suitable too, because the entrepreneurs have the ability to gather social resources to complete a large project. Dr. Yang are all of these, she is a female, a doctor, and an entrepreneur. I admire Dr. Yan's philanthropism, and, at the same time, I hope more and more people with multiple talents can join in this course, so that more people can be healthy early.

Case 16:

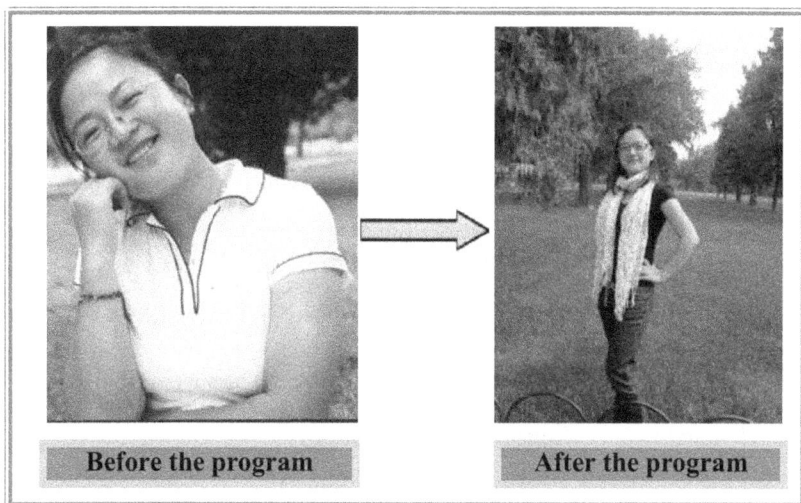

| Before the program | After the program |

I am Furong Jiang, and I am from Cixi, Zhejiang. I went to Beijing in 2001, and I am a housewife now. Since 2004, I had found myself depressed. Because every time when my husband went to work or went on business trip, after I sent my child to school, I had the kind of feeling that I was not needed, and I did not feel like doing anything. I thought that it was unnecessary to dress up while you were alone. I lied lazily on the sofa and watched TV, at the same time, I ate a lot of snakes. I hated to look in the mirror, because I felt disgusting when I looked at my body as it became round and big. I cheated myself by buying big and loose clothes because they can cover my big hip, and the 'life buoy' on my waist could not be easily seen. I rarely took photos of myself, and my temper became worse. I hated my current conditions, but I was very helpless, I didn't know how to change.

In August 2006, I was accompanied by my friend, Hongxian Wang, and started to learn about nutrition. I was lucky enough to be a student of Dr. Lu and became a practitioner of Dr. Lu's program.

After a cycle, I changed! My body shape and weight had changed by looking from the outside. From 59kg to 49kg, how amazing was this! Yet, I knew there was something more. I became happy, and had goals. When I was traveling to Malaysia in 2007, I was referred to as the 'Sunshine Angel', because I was just like a middle school student, but in fact, I was 34 years old that time, and a mother of a 7-year-old child. However, everyone said I was very young, and I was very happy. Since then, I fell in love with this program, and a strong sense of responsibility and mission arose spontaneously. I was eager to become a coach, and be a messenger to promote health. This decision has accompanied me until now, for eight years. Many things have happened over the past eight years, and I have experienced big changes in my life, but the only thing unchanged is the companion of this program.

I was 40 years old in 2014. People say that when you reached your forties, you will not be confused about life any more. However, I can only say I could not describe myself as happy, my heart was rather calm but joyful. I have obtained these after I decided to make changes. Because I am accompanied by this goal, my life is purposeful. I really feel like my life has begun to bloom like a flower.

Comments:

Furong represents a group of early practitioners. We advocate the use of lifestyle changes to solve lifestyle disease. Yet, in a stage that our theoretical system was not yet perfect, this group of people with their confirmation and long-term effective practice of this concept proved that lifestyle solutions to lifestyle disease was feasible. Not only is our short-term program effective, but the long-term program is also helpful. We cannot have completed the long, painful and happy transformation without the companion of this group of people.

Case 17:

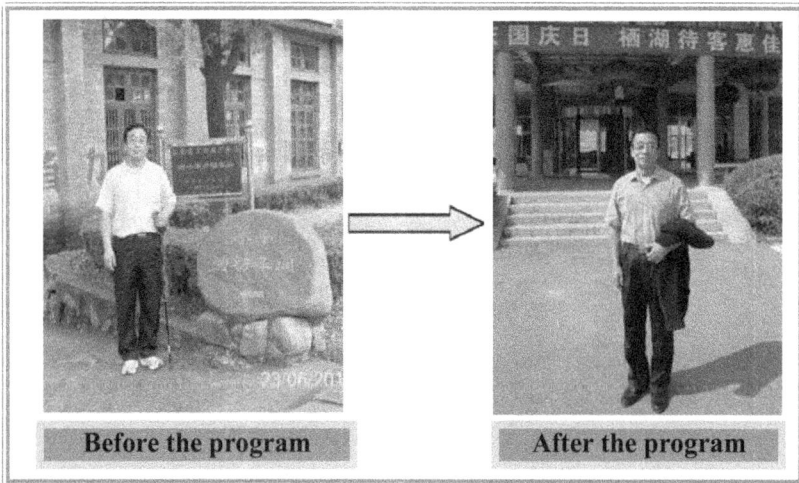

| Before the program | After the program |

Carrying out Doctor Lu's program, and allow health and wisdom to lead you to a happy life

My recovery benefits

(Qinglai Zhang, 61 years old, professor of International Education Management and Research, came back from Canada)

A healthy body and the method to live longer are always the ideal life journey for human kind. Yet I only truly understood the meaning of health when I luckily met Dr. Lu's program. At that time, my physical conditions were at their worst.

For a long time, due to inattention of health, coupled with an unhealthy lifestyle, my body had long been in a sub-health state. From time to time, my body sent out warning signals. As early as 2010, my right arm had part paralysis and movement disorders. In 2011, I had synovitis on my left knee and degenerative bone pain. My physical examination results showed that my weight was close to 100kg, which was seriously overweight. Lack of supply of blood and oxygen to my heart and brain had affected my memory and reflexes. Blood pressure reached 90mmhg-150mmhg, and I had moderate fatty liver. In addition, as many as thirteen indicators had problems, such as intraocular pressure, lipoprotein, uric acid etc. Although the signs had been so serious, but I had mistakenly believe that people would inevitably have some symptoms they when reached a certain age. I had no reason to stress out. So I did not take them seriously, so as that the development of various diseases became more and more severe.

At the end of 2012, under the sincere persuasion of medical research experts and friends, I took a try and participated in Dr. Lu's training camp. Through understanding and experiencing, I began to realize that I lacked self-awareness of my own health, and I ignored the correct way of life. I also realized that a healthy body came from cognition of health. Having the cognition of health meant that the person was smart and wise. The cognition was the base of a perfect life. Thus, I was firmly committed to the strict implementation of Doctor Lu's program.

Health miracle appeared! After a short period of intensified program, my weight dropped from 96kg to 79kg (reduced by 17kg), and high blood pressure also returned to 80-12 or so. The happiest thing was that after the weight loss, I had naturally stopped taking the daily drug for controlling blood pressure. Until today, my blood pressure has been kept normal. Knee pain, waist and leg pain and other limb pain have disappeared, and moderate fatty liver has also been converted to normal. I used to feel dizzy and sleepy, but now even I do not take a nap at noon, I feel energetic and can do fast walking. Friends say that I look like a different person.

As a direct beneficiary of Dr. Lu's program, I made an important choice regarding my career path. I would like to join the course of the program and continue to publicize and spread healthy ideas and healthy lifestyles, so that more friends can improve their health knowledge through our practice and health changes, and enhance the wisdom of life and health, so as to win a true sense of happiness in life.

Case 18:

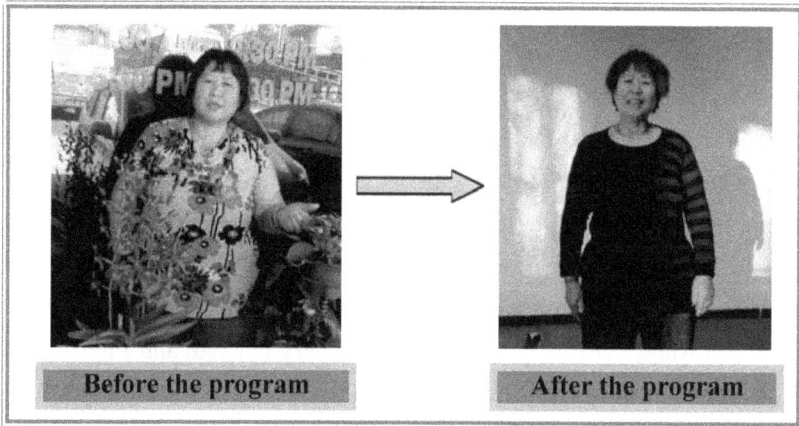

| Before the program | After the program |

My name is Xiulan Li and I am from Beijing. Below is my physical data before and after I took part in Doctor Lu's program:

	Before program	After program
Weight	110kg	75kg
BMI	39.5	25
Waist size	27	24

When I was young, I worked at a popsicle factory for more than 20 years. After getting old, it was too painful to walk. However, I still had to endure the pain every day. I went to the hospital for check-ups many times, also ate a lot of medicine, both Chinese and Western, but the pain did not become any better, and my husband had been taking care of me. Every time I saw my husband, I was thinking when could I stand on the ground, and personally make a meal for him? Yet, these had become a dream, and it was far away from me. When I saw my friends traveling, and participating in activities, I was very envious of them. I thought 'When can I travel and participate in activities with them?' Yet, I can only think.

By chance, an old friend came to my house to see me, and saw my painful looks and said, 'Your illness can be treated.' I heard but I was not happy. Because I did not believe that I would be so lucky, she was just saying to comfort me. A few days later, my friend called me, and started talking about my illness, and told me a lot of rehabilitated cases, but I still did not buy it. However, I really jealous of those people who had recovered from their illness, and I still hoped that such thing could happened to me. I discussed with my husband and decided to have a try.

In June 2013, I started the plan. My original weight is 110kg. I had been continuing the plan my coach gave me, and a week later I found that I lost 7.5kg. After two cycles of short-term intensive adjustment, my current weight is 75 kg. Now I can walk very relaxed, and I have a good mental state. I am very happy from the heart when I see the progress I have made.

Now I have been maintaining for a few months and there has been a very big change. My dream has come true. I can walk on my own, and occasionally, I can go travelling with my friends. I am ready to continue the program until my weight goes back to normal. I can also wear my favourite clothes, climb the mountain, feel the nature, and feel a better life!

Comments:

Obese people often accompanied by joint problems, the most common one is the degenerative arthritis of the knee joint, the other is the femoral necrosis. For such a phenomenon, the doctor will recommend the patient to lose weight, in order to reduce the burden on the body. Especially the knee, as the fulcrum of human movement, the load bearing ratio is 1: 6. If the part above your knee is 100 kg, when you go upstairs with force, the knee bears the weight of 600 kg. For obese people, the knee and hip joints wear faster than ordinary people. Through the intervention of the program, degenerative arthritis has been improved, and there is no longer 'creaky' sound, there is no need for the femoral head necrosis to replace the joints, why? There are two reasons, one is when the weight reduces, and knee fulcrum bears less pressure. If there was a weight loss of 10 kg, the pressure would be reduced by 60 kg; second, the program turns waste into wealth. Making the reduction of the 10 kg of fat transported to the cells, and the fat becomes the source of nutrition for human body rebuild, thus accelerating the knee and hip repair and self-healing, and bone density enhancement, periosteum regeneration and recovery.

Case 19:

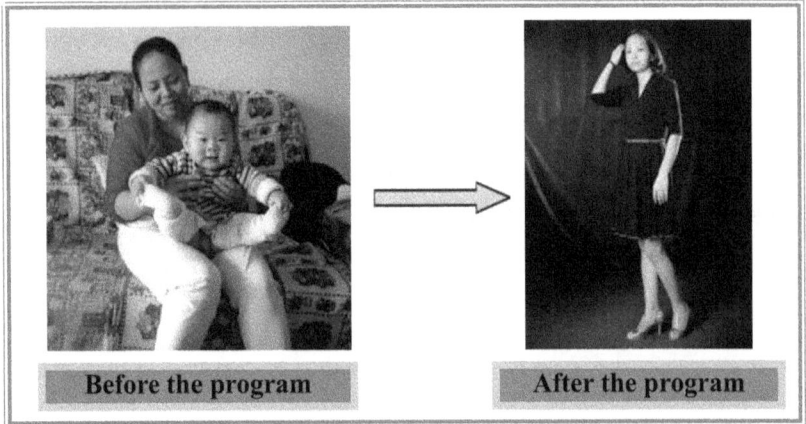

| Before the program | After the program |

My name is Yuan Yuan, 35 years old, mother of a two-year-old child. I did not have enough breast milk since my baby was born, so the child had been mixed feeding. Even so, when the child was almost 6 months, I did not have any breast milk to feed him. When he bit me with his 4 small teeth, I felt the pain in my heart, and I felt guilty. I really wanted to be a good mother, and brought him the best things in the world, but I did not have the ability to feed him. Watching my baby sleeping with tears and woke up crying, I had nothing but guilt and distress. Before this, in order to have more milk, I ate a lot every day, and my meal was equivalent two days of food of an adult, but my milk still reduced. When my baby was 6 months, I could not even squeeze out 20ml of milk. I was suffering from severe postpartum depression. I often looked out from the window of the 12th floor, and several times, I had the thought of jumping down, but I changed my mind when I thought of my baby's lovely face.

There were a few things which made me want to care about my own image. When my baby was 5 months old, I went to the shopping mall to buy clothes. The sales woman asked me with concern: 'When will you give birth?' I was so embarrassed to answer, 'I already have.' Another time when I took my baby home, and at the elevator, I met my neighbours.

They asked me curiously, 'The man who accompanies you every time, is he your younger brother?' But the man was actually my husband. I did not answer them but it really hurt my feelings. Every time when our family ate dinner together, my brother-in-law often asked me, 'When was the last time you look into the mirror? Aren't you afraid that you hundred will have an affair with another woman?' All the information made me realized how bad my situation was, and I made up my mind to make a change!

Finally, when the child was more than six months, I was lucky enough to have a phone conversation with Doctor Lu. After this, things changed. After two weeks of less intense adjustment, I suddenly found my breast milk thickened, when my baby was 7 months, he slept well after 10 minutes of breastfeeding, but before the program, he still cried after half an hour's breastfeeding. Since then, I had started breastfeeding until my baby was one year and four months old. At the same time I began to work and returned to normal diet. In one month, my weight reduced from 69.5kg to 50kg, and my body shape went back to the shape I was before I got pregnant. I am very grateful to Dr. Lu, he not only let me restore my body shape, but also let me restore the confidence in life, so that I have the ability to nurture a healthy baby.

Now I am like a happy little swallow, and have actively joined in the promotion of the program. I would like to share my own changes to all those who I know, and sincerely hope that my friends will meet Dr. Lu's program someday, and bring change to themselves and their family. I wish every friend to be healthy and happy!

Comments:

Ms. Yuan has solved the problem of postpartum milk shortage, and in the case of adequate milk, and the child is well-fed, her body recovered to the prenatal weight. Postpartum obesity and insulin resistance obesity are the same - metabolic disorders. Ms. Yuan ate a lot in the postpartum period, but there was no milk. So where were the foods that she had taken in? At this time, a lot of food is stored in the body in the form of fat, in subcutaneous, buttocks, and thighs, causing obesity, but produces no milk. A breast-feeding mother with normal metabolism should turn the things they eat into milk. Nowadays, mothers are fat, but lack of milk is a common phenomenon, which is mainly cause by metabolic problems. This program is a process of turning waste into wealth. Reusing the good things that they have consumed. When it is during the breastfeeding period, it is turned to milk. When it is during thinking, it is turned to brain power. When it is during exercising, it is turned into muscle power.

Case 20:

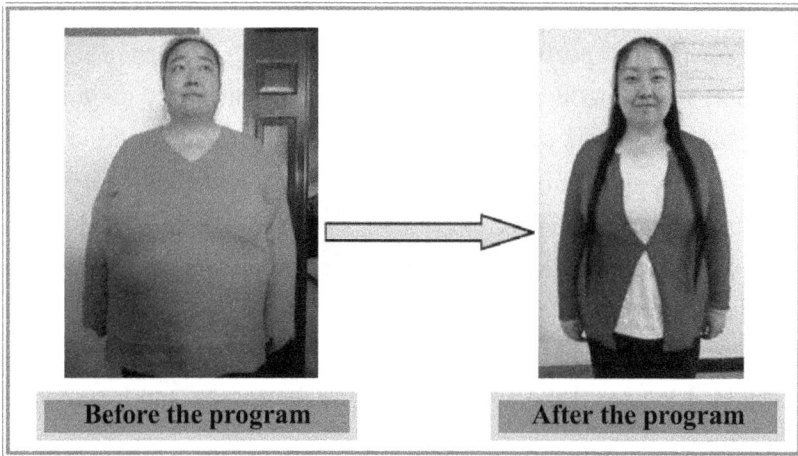

| Before the program | After the program |

My name is Mingyu Lu, female, 32 years old, I had participated in the program for 209 days.

I was fat since primary school, but I was not happy with obesity. From Junior high, I began to lose weight and had used lots of methods: weight loss biscuits, weight loss capsules, slimming tea, weight loss coffee, weight loss granular food, weight loss paste food; acupuncture, Chinese medicine, and running. I had tried all of the weight losing methods you could see in the market. Of course, there were side effects. I lost to 75kg once, but it rebounded and I became fatter. There is a good saying, the harder you try, the fatter you get. This is a summary of my years of trying. In 2012, due to work pressure, the elderlies at home were feeling unwell, coupled with hot summer weather, I often felt depressed and it was hard for me to walk. I was always sweaty and dizzy. I had long menstrual periods. I finally visited the doctor. At that time, my weight reached 125kg, I also had severe anaemia, 6 grams of haemoglobin, and there were obvious signs of diabetes - fasting blood glucose was more than 7 points, after dinner blood sugar reached around 12. Severe fatty liver, high uric acid also came to me. My menstrual period stayed for one month. This was really torture. Blood sugar and endocrine disorders forced me to stay in the hospital, my weight slightly decreased after I left hospital, but my conditions did not improve, I still needed to rest on bed when my menstrual period came. I went to see a Traditional Chinese doctor, and drunk more Traditional Chinese Medicine for more than six months, I ate donkey-hide gelatin, but the weight did not decrease, but rather, it increased from 125kg to 130kg. I was strengthless, I panted all the time, and I was unable to exercise, so most of the time I had to lie on the bed. I resigned from my work and stayed at home every day doing nothing. I felt psychological and physical stress. Seeing my classmates and friends had had their own business, and attended parties with their babies, I felt sad. I did not see where my future was, and I gave up my dreams.

In September 2013, my mother suddenly took home a set of health management program, after studying it for a while, she began to implement the program seriously every day. My father and I held a sceptical attitude, and once, we did not allow what my mother was doing. Yet, my mother did not listen to our advice, and insisted. In only one-month time, my mother had a significant change. Mom's migraine was completely cured, cervical pain for many years was solved, and her face became rosy, and her body became slim. These changes inspired me, and I decided to join the program.

At that time, my weight reached 132kg with severe fatty liver. Pale face, walking difficulty, endless menstrual period, and lying in bed all day, but under mother's supervision and accompany, and the guidance of my coach about my diet, water, exercise, sleep, urination, fat burning, etc., I was really touched, I was not fighting alone, everyone was working hard for me, and I shall not give up. After 209 days, my weight dropped to 95kg, by 37kg, and my face became rosy, my body had strength, and I had a good mood. Fasting blood sugar was at 5, the menstrual period became shorter. I felt, for the first time, that the sun was so bright, and full of hope. After weight loss, I walked every day for two hours without feeling tired. Now I have been engaged in this course, I am full of confidence and energy every day. My life has a purpose, and with hope. Health management is not just weight loss or stabilizing blood sugar, but it teaches you how to manage your own way of life and health, how to eat daily, from what you drink, exercise, and how you sleep etc. such small things to enhance the body's physical conditions. I think this are the worthiest gains.

Until today, I have lost 37kg, but it is only three-fifths of my goal. However, in the future, I will still be more confident. The two-fifths is not a daydream. I hope that my own experience can help everyone. Everyone is welcomed to continue to subscribe to my future changes. In the near future I will have a new change and you can see a beautiful me.

Comments:

Obesity not only destructs the body, but also the spirit, and even one who should have a happy life. A lot of obese people are debts of the society. They not only cannot create wealth, but also burden the family and society. This brings an unhealthy self-consciousness. Obesity people's weight loss struggle often end tragically, and it is detrimental to their personality and wills to fight. Eventually, they will not only give up losing weight, but also giving up the pursuit of a better life. The program is not only the reconstruction of the fat body, as well as their mind and life.

Case 21:

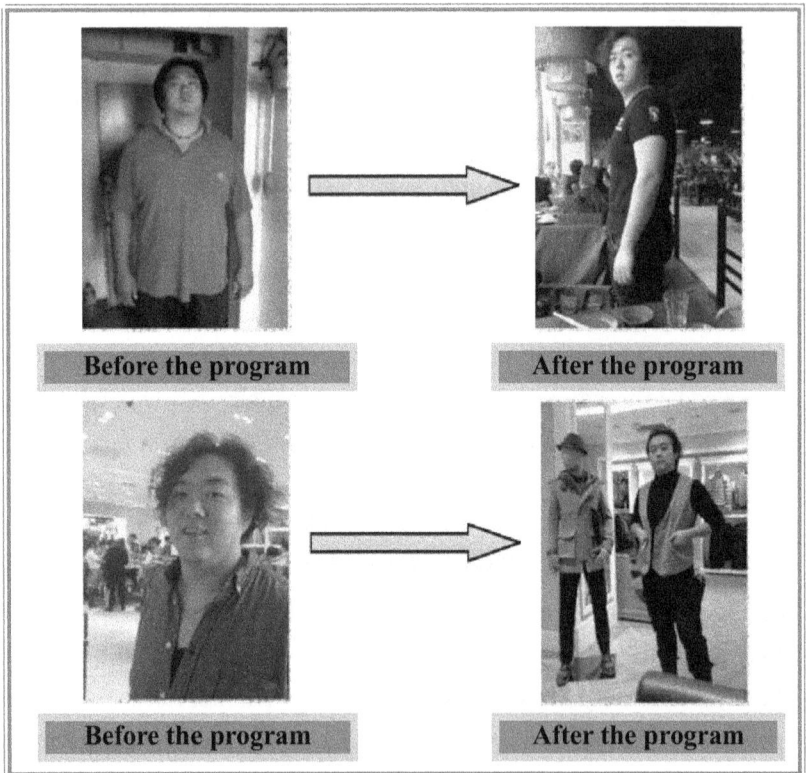

| Before the program | After the program |
| Before the program | After the program |

I am Li Bao, person-in-charge of a law firm in Beijing. I am 31 years old this year, my height is 188cm. My original weight was 135.5kg, now I weigh 119kg. I have spent half of my life losing weight. The weight always rebounded. No matter how good the methods were, my weight always rebounded. However, I never gave up. I entered the sprinting team at school when I was 10 years old. In junior high school, I changed to the basketball team. The, I entered the basketball team of a sports school. I had always exercised a lot. At that time, I was 182cm tall, and weighed 80kg, my body shape was pretty good. Then, in one of the practice competitions, I had a serious clash with someone, which severely damaged my ankles and my spine. After spending two months on bed resting, I gained 35kg. Moreover, there had been permanent damage to my spine. The doctor said, 'You will never be able to become an athlete. Don't forget to take breaks, you shouldn't have troubles to live an ordinary life.'

I thought I was dreaming, it was a blur when I accepted the truth of which I could not play basketball anymore. However, I thought some less intense exercises should have been fine. Yet, who knew, jogging for a short distance became impossible. At the start, I could not walk, run, or even sit, for too long. Just like this, I gradually stopped exercising. I put up a lot of weight, which burdened my spine. The more painful my spine was, the less exercises I could do. This created a vicious cycle.

Over these years, I tried every weight loss method as long as there had been success stories, I did not care if my weight would rebound, neither did I care about the sequelae the methods may bring. These methods included diet, exercise, oral administration, creams, acupuncture, and massages. In 2002, I used oral administration, diet and exercise at the same time. After three months, I lost 10kg. When I wanted to continue due to the confidence boost, the injuries kept hurting. Painkillers did not work. Thus, I had to stop trying to lose weight. Then we weight reached a record high: 140kg. Also, because I had been taking painkillers for too long, I had caffeine dependence. I had to drink lots of coffee every day, otherwise my headache would be so severe that I would not be able to fall asleep.

My mum recommended this program to me. I must admit, at the start, I was a bit sceptical. I had failed every time for 10 years, I had no hopes in losing weight. I implemented the program for the sake of my mum. The first three days, were like a nightmare. It was still awful even when I think of it now. It wasn't because of hunger, in fact, the program did not make me hungry at all. The nightmare was my caffeine dependence. My coach told me form the start that when I was using the program, the program would stimulate all of my diseases, and stimulate my instinct to self-heal the diseases, it may be painful. Although I had a brief idea, but I did not expect the extent. My head hurt so much that I felt like my eyes were going to pop out. I sweated so much that my shirt was soaked like it had been washed, yet I was cold. These feelings in one sentence were: I was going to die. Luckily, my parents and my partner kept comforting me, and my coach supported me, so I kept going on. Later in the program, there had been some pain in my back and legs, however they were nothing when compared to the headache. Just like this, I suffered for one week in hell.

From the second week and onwards, the uncomfortableness disappeared. I was 0.5kg lighter every morning. The feeling was very good. By the way, I had never drank coffee ever since that day.

After two cycles, my weight reduced from 235.5kg to 103kg. Weight wise, I lost 32.5kg, waist size wise, it went from 110cm to 88cm. I did not drink any more coffee, my stomach did not hurt anymore. The lumber calcification, which I had had for 20 years, did not hurt anymore. The feeling was really good, I cannot put them into words.

Afterwards, I have summarized my weight loss experience, and arrived at a conclusion: attitudes are very important. Everyone must have a positive attitude, not only for the sake of losing weight. Don't give up on yourself ever. I have learnt how to comfort myself. Do not give yourself too much pressure. Through this experience, I believe that I can do anything I want to. I really like this phrase from a movie, 'Who said there was no shortcuts in losing weight? When you find the correct method, and you are not off track, then that is the shortcut.'

Comments:

When implementing our program, sometimes people can successfully get rid of caffeine or tobacco addiction. Why can a weight loss program help to get rid of addictions? This is because the program helps with the restoration of human instinct.

Human brains can secrete substances which make people feel happy, safe and accomplished. These substances are called 'happiness hormone'. For example, 'dopamine' which brings happiness, 'norepinephrine' which brings passion, 'endorphin' which kills pain, and 'oxytocin' which helps us to overcome obstacles.

Most of the time, only a little bit of happiness hormones is secreted, which keeps us calm. Only when we achieve our goals, the brain would secrete more happiness hormones as a reward, making us feel contented and happy, and take away mental and physical pain which may negatively influence us. The harder and the bigger the goal is, the more happiness hormones are secreted. This type of response reinforces those positive actions which promote the secretion of happiness hormones. This type of instinct is a thoughtful design, allowing humans to face challenges, overcome hardships, and improve the society.

'Addiction' is when humans use drugs to 'steal' happiness hormones, which causes the body to not be able to get the same amount of happiness hormones through ordinary lifestyles. The more drugs are used for longer, human functions degenerate more. When we leave the addictions, we may feel uncomfortable, like emptiness, depression, or even headaches, diarrhoea, muscle spasm, and convulsion. This results in addiction (because we cannot leave them)

This program aims to restore human instinct. When humans can discrete happiness hormones normally, the dependence on the addictions will decrease.

Case 22:

Hello everyone, I am Yonghong Zhao, from Shilou Province, Lvliang Suburb, Shanxi State. I am 38 years old this year. I had been fat ever since I was young. I had been fat for half of my life. The pain could not be put into words, people who had never been fat before could never understand the pain.

At my heaviest, I was 180kg. I could not take care of myself. I could not wash my face or feet. I had tried more than 20 weight loss methods, but they all failed. After losing weight, I had not yet enjoyed the happiness, I quickly regained weight again. I regained 5 to 10kg every time. My waist size increased 7cm every time. The more I tried to lose, the more I gained.

This May, I went to Taiyuan to meet my teacher. I could not kneel to bow to my teacher. It was difficult to stand up again after kneeling down. When I left, my teacher gave me some materials, and told me that his student, Yongna Fei was promoting the program. My teacher thought the program may be helpful for me. Yet, I did not care about it that much because I had given up on losing weight. However, as a student, I took the materials home for the sake of respecting my teacher. I had a read in my free time. From my experience, I thought the book was quite reasonable, and gave a lot of insights. The explanations were also scientific. I read it three times, and I thought the plan was doable.

After a few days, I went to Taiyuan to see my senior – Yongna Pei. This was to understand the program further. On June 1st, I went to the training camp based in Beijing, and started to implement the program. The results were much better than I expected. I am telling the truths; the program is actually incredible! In three months of intensified short-term plan, my weight decreased from 161.5kg to 112.5kg. Other data were: my waist size decreased from 132cm to 100cm. I had nail fungus on all ten toes. Now, four of them had healed completely, and the other six were half way through healing. My Comprehensive Metabolic Panel data were: uric acid from 738.7 to 519.8; low-density lipoprotein went from 3.76 to 3.52; triglyceride decreased from 1.48 to 1.4; and my fasting blood glucose went from 5.97 to 5.68. I am still implementing the program, I will continue this until I reach my ideal weight. This method is so good, it is so easy to continue it! I now have started to promote and advertise this program. This program can bring people health and help the nation. If I do so, I will also feel happy and sense of accomplishment.

Comments:

After the program, Mr. Zhao's nail fungi were improved. Nail fungus is considered as one of the hardest diseases to cure. Why is this plan useful when curing nail fungus? This is because nail fungus is an autoimmune disease, it is caused by infections of fungi. Infections often occur when the immunity of one is weak. For autoimmune diseases, we can eliminate the diseases by improving our immunity system. Psoriasis, hepatitis B, and such diseases, can be improved after implementation of the program, because these diseases are all autoimmune diseases.

Chapter Two: Practice Instruction

I. Five Advices for the Public

In order to live healthier and for longer, we not only need to exploit the wisdom of cells, but also, we have become smarter regarding health. The following five health insights are the most important mental fundaments to be healthy in real life.

1. Where there is life, there is hope

Modern scholars have had intensive researches on 'Sun Tzu's Art of War', and they have reached a surprising conclusion: 'The highest state of military is not to win, but not to lose'. Where there is life, there is hope. As long as you have not lost, there is a chance to win. As long as you have not lost, you can win. The same as life. If one is healthy, everything is possible. Loss of health is losing everything. 'The body is the capital of revolution'. For everyone, health is the capital for pursuing personal growth and development, managing family and career, and becoming wealthier. Health is the core assets of life, managing health is to manage family and career, and managing health is managing happiness and joy. The person who laughs till the end may not be the richest, but they must be healthiest and longest-living. Arthur Schopenhauer, a German Philosopher, pointed out that 'The greatest of follies is to sacrifice health for any other kind of happiness.› Bible says ‹And what do you benefit if you gain the whole world but lose your own soul? Is anything worth more than your soul?

2. Preparedness ensures success, and unpreparedness spells failure

Preparedness ensures success, and unpreparedness spells failure. Same applies to maintaining health. The prevention before illness is better than treatment after illness, and daily health care is better than temporary exercise. A wise man will prevent illness even when he is healthy, which allows him to live longer. A normal man will go to see a doctor after getting the disease, and he would feel fatigue in his fifties. A fool man will not care about diseases, whether big or small, then he would eventually have to spend money for health, and die at an early age. The modern medicine shows that the natural human life span is fixed, and cannot be extended. The Chinese traditional medicine also believes that the chi (vigour) that people is born with is limited. It cannot increase, it can only decrease. If the chi is not completely exhausted, people would still have a spark of life left; if it is exhausted, any method is useless. So, people cannot extend lifespan, but they can save chi, reduce loss of chi, and live as long as they are destined to be. The economists point out that maintaining health is an investment with the greatest return. The important economic conclusion informs us that we should pay lots of attention to health, maintain health and invest in health even when we are very healthy.

The greatest health insight is to be prepared for danger while we are still safe. Treating disease when getting sick is like 'fixing the fence after a sheep is lost' (meaning 'too late'). Getting an illness will shorten one's lifespan, and the shortened life span cannot be recovered. Simiao Sun could live to 141, this did not rely on 'fixing the fence after a sheep is lost', but being prepared for danger in times of safety. Only we have crisis awareness, we can cherish health, actively learn and take positive actions while we are still healthy. It is very easy to be carried out in dribs and drabs at anytime from anywhere.

3. Contentment and gratefulness

Happy people do not age, because happiness is the best medicine. The extent of happiness of one depends on one's contentment and gratefulness. The senior statesman of the Republic of China (1921-1949), Mr. Youren Yu, had been through the miserable vicissitudes of life but lived to 86. Friends asked him for the way to keep in good health. He pointed to the antithetical couplet in the living room, and smiled silently.

The first line was 'Do not think about undesirable things'; the second line was 'Always think about happy things'; streamer was 'As you wish'.

Sigh about undesirable things in the life; and often think about happy things, you will be smiling all the time, and keep yourself open-minded and carefree. If heart is driven by materials, and swayed by considerations of gain and loss, the mind will only be stifled by pessimism and desperation. One will struggle in life, even, damage the body and shorten the lifespan.

4. Health lies in habits

Habit is the outline of health, and when it is laid out, the details are easy to deal with. 'Habits are the secrets that can only be understood by a few wise men'. Two weaknesses of life restrict us from obtaining health: first, we know what to do but we do not do them; second, we sometimes do them but we do not continue doing them. Regarding health, we become healthy because of habits, but we also become unhealthy because of habits.

Habits need to be deliberately established. When bad habits are being replaced with good habits, temporary uncomfortableness can occur. The uncomfortableness is the cause of more failures of establishing a good habit. So, the key of establishing good habits is to overcome temporary uncomfortableness. According psychology, a habit can be formed if it is repeated every day for 21 days. Both good habits and bad habits will affect our life unconsciously. So, developing habits is the real solution that is useful forever. Managing habits is the best strategy to manage health.

5. Health lies within simplicity

There are many factors which affect health. Yet, there must be a significant and a not so significant effect on health. Simplicity is to make a distinction between the significant and the less significant one. To be able do the simplest thing is to be able to do the most important thing. The simpler the health program, the greater the chance of continuing it for a lifetime. It is meaningless to do any better regimen for a short time.

Make the three simplest things as your habits, and then the lifestyle disease will have nothing to do with you for a lifetime:

Give priority to coarse food for the staple food;

Continue to supplement trace elements;

Combination of exercise and meditation.

II. Three Instructions for the Coach

(Selective reading for patients, compulsory reading for practitioners)

If you decide to devote yourself to this program, then you will become a coach. The denotative coach is the professional that provides one-to-one health guidance. The connotative coach is the coach leader who organizes a coach team to guide a large group of crowds.

Being a coach is meaningful. What you bring for the people is not just health, you will change their lives, change a family, a tribe, even a nation. The world will change because of you, and will be more beautiful because of you.

Good things start with establishing our own identity. Firstly, we need to establish good thoughts, purifying the hearts, then cultivate the body. Eventually, the family will live in harmony, the country will be strong, and the world will be united.

The following are our three great basic beliefs. We hope that you, as a coach, can acknowledge them. We believe that you and I not only are able to meet in the journey, but also are likely to go together with these consensuses.

1. Be your best

Humans are born with meanings. The most meaningful life is when the gifts of people are exploited to the greatest extent possible, and the world becomes more wonderful.

Make a greater contribution to society by being better; and be better through the greater contributions. The best way to maximize contribution is to explore the one's potentials and gifts to the utmost extent. Do your best, then you can live the most meaningfully.

If one is born as a tree, then live out the height and straightness of tree, and make the mountains appear to look better. One is born as a flower, then live out the gorgeousness of a flower, and make world more colourful. If one is born as grass, then live out the vibrancy of the grass, and make the ground more elegant. Be whoever you are; what gift you are endowed with, then live out your talents. Make the world more beautiful than it ever has been by being the best of yourself.

2. Passion is the mother of success

The attitudes decide everything. Attitudes decide if one is ordinary or extraordinary. Many positive attitudes help us to become good coaches. The most significant and crucial one is 'passion'.

Bill Gates dropped out when he was a sophomore, the most moving reason for it is 'I only feel good when I sit in front of a computer'. Not the desire of making money, but the passion for technology, created the youngest and richest man in the world. Jordan retired three times, every return of him is not to make more money, but he just can't help but to carry on and cherish it. It is not the ambition which makes a fortune, but the raging passion creates the greatest sports stars and the richest tale in the sports circles in human history.

Passion is the most powerful strength in the world. The difference between the ordinary and the extraordinary is the passion. The accumulation of knowledge is in dribs and drabs, and the growth of mind is by leaps and bounds, and the greatest driving force for tremendous growth is passion. There are many teachers in our life, and the best one is passion. Potential is the largest gold mine in life, and passion is the most effective tool for exploring potential. There are many definitions of success, the most eloquent one is 'success if when you do what you like with all you might'. There are many roads that lead to success, and the most beautiful road is passion. The people who success due to passion forget themselves, and welcome the embrace of success in the process of enjoying life bloom.

The whole meaning of a match coming to the world is to ignite for one time. Burning itself is not only to illuminate others, but also to light others up, and illuminate the world.

You only live once, you should love your life, ignite yourself, and be beautiful. If you would like to be an excellent coach, then be passionate about the program.

3. Love is action, action is a gain

In a heavy snow night in winter, a girl comes home from school with a bag on the back, walks to the doorway, and sees that a dog, near the door, is crouching in the corner and shaking. The girl opens the door and rushes to mom's embrace, and says that, 'Mom, the dog in the doorway is really pitiful!' Whereas, under the same circumstances, that a boy sees the same dog, runs to home and says to his mother, 'Mom, the dog in the doorway is really pitiful. Can I share half of my dinner with it?' What the story tells is that love is action.

There are three frogs standing on a lotus leaf, and one of them wants to jump down. How many frogs are left on the lotus leaf? Three. There are three frogs left. That frog is only thinking, and nothing happens. No action? No love.

What the action is a gain tells is not 'no pain, no gain', neither is 'virtue has to be its own reward'. What it does tell is that what we do currently is a gain. Because you have done that thing, then you become a person with fuller heart, a happier soul and a more elegant life. As the extremely beautiful phrase stated – 'Love, will never disappoint you. Love will always flow back to your heart to warm you and purify your soul, even though it does get anything in return.

III. Extraordinary Characteristics of Leaders of the Industry

(Selective reading for patients, compulsory reading for practitioners)

Any era has its own problems. If we devote ourselves into solving the problem, then we have the opportunity of solving it. The best way to promote the evolution of the society is to be the best of ourselves. Lifestyle disease is the product of modern civilization, and it also provides an unprecedented industry opportunity for the people born in this era.

The health industry serves as the promising rising industry. Its development meets the fundamental requirements of human, and the health industry will be the industry which supports the nation's economy. The data shows that, currently, health service industry only accounts for about 5 % of GDP in China, and the same industry in America reached up to 17.6% in 2009. The wave of high-tech revolution has been turned from IT technology to HT industry (health industry). The health industry contributes more than 10% of GDP in Canada, Japan and other countries. The developed countries have the health industry as the strategic focus of the economic and social developments. For example, Japan has listed the health industry and new energy, energy-saving and environment-friendly industries, as the strategic focus of future economic development.

China, with 1.3 billion people, working as a big country from median-income country to a country with high-income, the health industry is very likely to expand in the future. According to a survey of China Merchants Bank in 2011, among the requirements of value-added service of high-net-worth individuals (with more than 10 million investable assets), the medical health service accounted for 44%, which was over the 'children's education' and 'introduction of investment opportunity'. Health service has risen to be the first requirement of the crowd. According to the calculations of the authority, the total scale of China's healthcare industry will reach as high as over 8 trillion CNY (approx. $1.1 trillion USD) by 2020. The flourishing health industry will be new growth point of China's national economy.

In the new field, we are on the same level as developed countries, we are standing on the same starting line. The lifestyle disease is a common new topic that human face. When internet appeared as a new thing, we were on the same level as the developed countries. When Google and Facebook have appeared in America, the giants: Tencent, Baidu and Alibaba, which have the scale over one hundred million CNY (approx. 14 million USD) or even one trillion CNY ($136 USD) have appeared in China. What make people amazed is that all of these only take more around ten years. In the next ten or even twenty years, what steps onto the historical stage is health industry. The trend shows that new giants of the economy are being created. Chinese health industry will grow spectacularly. The government has force some national, or even global brands, such as the well-known Haier and Midea, in the household appliance industry, Lenovo and Huawei in the IT industry, and Tencent, Baidu and Alibaba of the internet industry.

The great attention from the government to health industry will accelerate the release of the great potential of China's health industry. On August 28, 2013, Premier Keqiang Li presided executive meeting of the state council to discuss, and lay out policies and measures to encourage the development of the healthcare industry. The meeting emphasized the need to fully initiate the social power and accelerate it to develop content-rich and multilevel healthcare industry, which was effectively protect basic medical and health service requirement of the masses. The meeting pointed out that in order to promote the development of healthcare industry, the focus is to increase supply; the core is to ensure quality; and the key is to rely on reformation and innovation.

The major problem of healthcare industry, is that, at the present stage, the contradiction between the growing demand for health of human and the relatively decreasing industry supply. The key to solve the problem neither lies in increasing production capacity, nor lies in improving the service level. Rather, it lies in increasing effective supply. Expanding effective supply will bring not only the massive improvement of people's health, but also the flourishing development of the industry.

In the next ten years, or the next twenty years, what kinds of enterprises can be the industry leader or the new giants? It must not be the mediocre ones who pursue profits. The remarkable achievement must belong to the enterprises with a primitive desire and a want beyond profits, which mainly focuses on the health and longevity of people. The enterprises that have achieved temporary success today can only achieve the development from extraordinary to even more outstanding as long as they finish the growth of the mind. It is not important if the enterprise is big. The dinosaurs were big, but they could not withstand the change of environment. In an era when everything is changing, the dinosaur that lived the best had never been the biggest one, even not the strongest, but the one that adapted to the era the most. God helps those who comply with the way of living according to God. 'The way of heaven is to benefit others and not to injure'. The way of how enterprises survive and develop rests on adapting social development and promoting social progress. The nature of the enterprises is to organize unordered resources (including labour, land, and capital and such etc.) to solve the problems which cannot be done by only one man. The bigger the problem, the more successful the enterprise is. Profit is the by-product of value, and the best way to make profit is to create value. Without creating the value, no matter how good the profit model is, it will be at best a flash in the pan.

Conclusion
-- Further Discussion on 'Solving Lifestyle Disease with Lifestyle'

The essence of lifestyle disease is the problem of modern civilization. In addition to how the modern civilization has made our life richer and more convenient, the modern civilization also forces humans to be far away from nature, and makes life to deviate from its original will. The phenomenon is called as the 'alienation of civilization' in philosophy. Human encounters extensive lifestyle disease with the development to modern civilization. Historically, this phenomenon is inevitable.

We do not deny how the modern civilization has put forward 'Solving Lifestyle Disease with Lifestyle'. We also do not advocate living in seclusion and cultivating by ourselves. I did not propose that in a small country with a small population and everyone should be completely isolated from each other for the rest of their lives. It is not bad, but it just is that not all of 7 billion people cannot do it. The retrogression and inaction of civilization cannot solve the problems that human encounter in the development of civilization.

What 'solving lifestyle disease by lifestyle' advocates are to solve the problem encountered in the process of development with further development, and address the challenges the modern civilization faces by higher civilization. On the one hand, comply with social development, comply with the inevitable trends that human materialized civilization is becoming richer and richer, and the spiritual civilization is more and more developed. We enjoyed the abundant internet brought by the modern civilization, and made use of the convenience provided by the achievement of modern civilization. On the other hand, comply with nature, including complying with the nature that has been changed due to human activities, and also including complying with the original will of life.

The society is developing, and humankind is also improving. So, the modern civilization characterized by industrial civilization and information civilization will be replaced by higher-level civilization. The higher-level civilization should be much more developed, meanwhile, we should comply with nature better. We do not know how the people will name the civilization in the future. It may be ecological civilization, or nature civilization. Yet, no matter what they name it, the higher-level civilization must meet the most important standards: make humans happier, and make the world more beautiful.

www.ingramcontent.com/pod-product-compliance
Lightning Source LLC
Chambersburg PA
CBHW020658270326

41928CB00005B/180